Preface

Anyone who studies history will be able to speak to the singularity of 'in-vogue' phenomena, concepts, and/or behaviours; and the history of nursing (or perhaps more accurately nursing science) is no exception. This notion of being 'in vogue' captures the idea that some things are said to be in accordance with current 'social' fashions or trends; or in the case of nursing, in accordance with nursing fashions or trends. One could construct a cogent case today in 2009 that one such in-vogue concept in nursing is 'evidence-based' (or more accurately 'evidence-informed') practice. In the UK in the 1980/90s it could be suggested that the so-called 'nursing process' was then the 'in-vogue' idea. Another phenomenon that might be so categorised (perhaps more so in the USA) could be the so-called 'nursing diagnosis'. It seems that concepts, practices and phenomena such as these become an integral part of the everyday parlance of nurses and nursing; although it also seems to be the case that the 'timespan' of being the in-vogue concept of the day is always limited. It is difficult to examine the history of nursing without seeing evidence that nursing models once occupied the position of being the in-vogue concept of the day, although it is equally accurate to purport that the halcyon days of nursing models are behind us.

It has often been pointed out that nursing models and nursing theory are of limited value if they do not influence practice, and practice without theory is baseless. (Here the authors deliberately conflate the terms nursing theory and nursing models, although we acknowledge and recognise that some nurse theorists would not agree with this stance.) It is therefore surprising that many clinical nurses in the 21st century still do not see the importance of nursing theories. It was not always so, as we pointed out above; there are arguably at least two periods of time in the history of nursing when nursing models were in vogue. In the 1950/60s and then again in the 1980s such models were appreciated, analysed and applied. They underpinned care plans and curricula. However, they were often imposed by managers and implemented rigidly and bureaucratically. These may be some of the reasons why clinical nurses today place less value on nursing models. Whatever the reasons, it is evident that they did indeed appear to 'fall out of favour' (just as all in-vogue concepts do).

However, the authors of this book argue that wholesale rejection of nursing models is problematic at best and deleterious to the discipline of nursing at worst. Yet creating another book that examines nursing models, in a climate where they are not currently in vogue; and when there are already in existence some fine examples of scholarly works that appear to focus on the theoretical dimensions of nursing models, would seem the height of folly. Therefore this book deliberately and purposefully adopts a different emphasis. The authors believe that this book can help revitalise the centrality of nursing theories/models for patient care. It does this by showing how models can influence the way nurses think and act and how the care of patients, their families and communities can be enhanced as a result. Most especially, while acknowledging and valuing the theoretical underpinnings and origins of nursing models, the book focuses on the application of nursing models in clinical practice. Given that nursing is a pragmatic, practice-orientated discipline, it is in such application that the value and utility of nursing models are best experienced.

John Cutcliffe
Hugh P. McKenna
Kristiina Hyrkäs

Foreword

Callista Roy, PhD, RN, FAAN

The demands of the 21st century challenge nurses to use knowledge to contribute to the health of individuals and the good of society. As a discipline nursing has made great strides in recent decades in knowledge-based practice as theoretical frameworks were developed to guide practice and research. Good, up-to-date literature that reflects these developments makes an important contribution to the use of knowledge in practice. This book makes a significant contribution to the available literature. First, it is a fresh conceptualisation of a book on nursing models. It initially offers a clear and direct discussion of what models are, which can be useful for the neophyte who does not have this background or for the experienced scholar searching for the words to articulate the meaning and significance of nursing models. Higher level concepts such as paradigms are explained and integrated into the reader's understanding. A brief history provides a context for appreciating the work that has gone before and the challenges that lie ahead.

Secondly, it is a privilege to introduce this book because the design of the chapters allows for in depth applications to many areas of nursing practice. By selecting seven major models the authors succeed in describing and critiquing each model in sufficient detail and clarity for both beginners and advanced readers. By limiting the number of models covered, it is possible to go into depth both on the theoretical application to practice and to give case studies as well as pertinent literature reviews of use of the model in practice as well as in research. The authors provide a teaching instrument that is greatly needed in nursing education in both academic and clinical settings. They have managed to provide the emphasis that is needed to move theory-based practice to a new level.

The chapter authors as a group have responded to the challenge of taking a broad theoretical perspective on nursing practice for individuals, families, and communities. At the same time the details of specific theoretical approaches are addressed. The reader obtains a more comprehensive view of theory-based practice by comparing how each model approaches given clinical situations in settings from the hospital to the home and community. The authors handle issues of different healthcare systems and different cultures in a straightforward manner so that the flow of thought is not interrupted. The work can provide the basis for highlighting the role of nurses in interdisciplinary team approaches to the increasingly complex health challenges of our time.

Foreword

Alison J. Tierney, PhD, FRCN, CBE

It is a privilege to have the Roper-Logan-Tierney model for nursing, with which I am connected, included, along with six other well-known nursing models, in this book. It is now nearly a decade since I worked with the late Nancy Roper and our colleague Win Logan to write the monograph that provides a final account of our model, published in the year 2000, exactly 20 years after its original launch in *The Elements of Nursing* (1980). Over the years, this book went through several new editions, it was translated into many different languages, and our model became widely known around the world. Although we now leave others to use and develop our model in ways they find appropriate and helpful, it is still exciting to come across new references to our work.

It takes skill to produce a book that at one level is suitable for nursing students at the beginning of their studies and yet, at another, has sufficient depth and detail to satisfy more advanced students and even experienced practitioners. Each of the chapters that focuses on a particular model starts with a brief history of that model and a profile of the person/s who developed it. Then, in describing each model and analysing its essential parts, the authors draw on the opening chapters in which the nature of nursing models and nursing theory are dissected and discussed. These opening chapters are, in their own right, valuable, but their underpinning of each of the model chapters – and the iteration of nursing's metaparadigm concepts – is one of the great strengths of the book. Each of the model chapters is brought to a close with examples and/or case studies to demonstrate application of the model and a review of contemporary literature pertaining to the model, the latter providing evidence of its clinical, empirical and theoretical impact.

However, the real challenges, for the authors of this book and for its readers, come in the final chapter, which addresses the question of how a nursing model can be critiqued. The ideas of the late 1980s and early 1990s for the evaluation of nursing models are still pertinent, in particular the ideas and framework developed by Jacqueline Fawcett. However, the authors of this book recognise that evaluation of nursing models now needs to be reconsidered in the contemporary context in which the concept of evidence-based practice has come to dominate nursing and healthcare. At the same time, as the authors describe, there is now a much wider range of research methodologies available for the purpose of evaluation, including the mixing of quantitative and qualitative methods. These advancements in research should be used to advantage, this book argues, in any contemporary evaluation of nursing models.

Acknowledgements

John Cutcliffe: I am indebted to the unswerving support of my wife Maryla and my family.
This book is dedicated to my first daughter, Natalia Faith, who brings added meaning to life. It is also dedicated to the instructors, authors, peers and students who have discussed and debated matters related to nursing models – you have my most profound thanks.

Kristiina Hyrkäs: This book is dedicated to my family, colleagues and to those nurses whose insightful observations and questions have stimulated my writings about nursing theories and models in practice.

Hugh McKenna:I would like to acknowledge the unstinting support of my wife Tricia, my son Gowain and my daughter Saoirse. I would also like to thank the many students whose perceptive questions over the years have had the desired ripple effect in developing my thinking about nursing models and theories.

To Sister Callista Roy and Alison Tierney we offer our deepest gratitude not only for the fine forewords you kindly provided, but for your seminal contributions to nursing science.

To Jessica Anderson, whose copy editing made this process very enjoyable and to Maria Anguita, whose patience and guidance have been invaluable, we thank you.

John Cutcliffe is currently an Adjunct Professor at the University of Ulster (UK), and the University of Malta; most recently he held the 'David G. Braithwaite' Endowed Professorial Chair of Nursing at the University of Texas (Tyler), USA.

He has written more than 150 papers and eight books and has over $4 million of extra-mural research funding as Primary/Co-Investigator. In 2003 he was recognised by the Federal Government of Canada and cited as one of the top 20 'Research Leaders of Tomorrow' for his research focusing on hope and suicidology. In 2004, he was nominated for a Canadian Research Chair in Suicidology and was given the highest research rating, 'outstanding', from the independent reviewers. He has recently served as the national Canadian Representative for the International Association of Suicide Prevention and the Director of the International Society of Psychiatric Nurses: Education and Research Division: he is also an Assistant Editor for the *International Journal of Nursing Studies* and an Associate Editor for the *International Journal of Mental Health Nursing*.

Hugh McKenna is a Professor and Dean at the University of Ulster and he holds several adjunct appointments.

He has over 200 publications including nine books and over £2.5 million in grants. He has supervised 14 PhD students to successful completion and chaired the UK Government's assessment of nursing. He has also researched, taught and written on nursing theories and models. He is an editor of the *International Journal of Nursing Studies* and has received many prestigious awards including Fellow of the Royal College of Nursing, Fellow of the European Academy of Nursing, Fellow of the Royal College of Surgeons of Ireland, International Fellow of the American Academy of Nursing, and Commander of the British Empire (CBE).

Both John Cutcliffe and Hugh McKenna are currently working with colleagues from Dublin City University and the University of Toronto on an international programme of research focusing on suicide, more specifically on suicide following discharge and suicide in young men. They have a number of future collaborations planned with regard to mental health nursing and on-line learning.

Kristiina Hyrkäs is at present Director of the Center for Nursing Research and Quality Outcomes at Maine Medical Center, Portland, Maine, USA. She is also an Adjunct Professor of Nursing at the University of Southern Maine, College of Nursing and Health Professions.

She is currently supervising three PhD students and many hospital-based research, quality improvement and evidence-based practice projects. She is one of the editors for the *Journal of Nursing Management*, and an editorial board member for another international journal.

She co-chairs the publication committee of the International Network for Doctoral Education in Nursing and reviews manuscripts for 12 academic journals using three different languages. She has published 50 articles in peer reviewed journals, nine book chapters and four books.

CHAPTER I

What are nursing models and why do we need them?

At the outset, and in order to understand subsequent chapters, it would be good to get rid of some of the confusion around terminology. As readers you will often come across the following terms in the nursing literature: conceptual framework, theory, model, phenomena, concepts, propositions, and many others. In the next few paragraphs we will clarify the more common terms and this should provide you with a platform to understand and appreciate the rest of the book.

How are models/theory constructed?

In everyday practice you will come across interesting events or happenings. For instance, you may see a patient giving information to another patient after the latter has been given a similar diagnosis. This is something you experience through your senses – in this case sight and hearing. What you are noticing is called a phenomenon. Meleis (1991: 201) stated that: 'When experience and sensory and intuitive data become coherent as a whole, and prior to any attachment of meaning, we have a phenomenon.'

Models in ancient times

It is our view that the development of all models and theories starts with someone noticing a phenomenon. Why is it happening? How is it happening? What has to be in place for it to happen? The history of the world and our most important discoveries can be traced to people asking these questions about phenomena they come across.

We include three examples from a very large list: In ancient Greece, Archimedes from Syracuse (c.287BC–c.212BC) noticed that when he was taking a bath his body displaced bathwater. From this he theorised that a body immersed in a fluid experiences a buoyant force equal to the weight of the displaced fluid. From this he developed a buoyancy theory and with further testing this phenomenon was known as the Archimedes principle.

In the middle ages, Galileo Galilei (1564–1642) invented the telescope. He noticed that the earth appeared to go around the sun and not the other way round. This got him into trouble with the church who preached that the earth was the centre of the universe. He was placed under arrest and it took hundreds of years before the church posthumously forgave him. More recently, Charles Darwin (1809–1882) noticed that extinct species were preserved in fossils. From this he presented to the world his theory of evolution. This got him into trouble with the church too, and it still does.

What these scientists discovered and started to notice over long periods of time were phenomena. They took an interest in these phenomena and with further work they ended up with the buoyancy, heliocentric and evolutionary theories. As with Galileo, Archimedes and Darwin we all notice phenomena throughout our daily lives but on most occasions we do not pay much attention to them – so new knowledge is often lost.

In addition, Archimedes was able to explore his theory through the use of a hydrometer and Galileo was only able to set out his theory because he had discovered the telescope. So too, novel technologies in healthcare uncover many new phenomena that await our attention.

Phenomena to concepts to propositions to models and theories

But how do you move from phenomena to models? We will give you an example. Let's say that over a period of time you notice that patients who have urinary incontinence have difficulty talking about sexuality or indeed they tell you that they have no interest in establishing or maintaining sexual relationships. Here you are noticing a phenomenon through your senses of hearing and seeing. Of course, as with most phenomena, you could ignore it. However, on this occasion you decide to check if this is something that others have noticed. So you mention this to other nurses and they too have had similar experiences with patients who have urinary incontinence. You also review the literature to see if this is something that is commonly highlighted or researched. However, after a comprehensive search, you cannot find any mention of it.

The next step is to name or put a label onto what you have noticed. When you do this you are creating a concept, for a concept is simply a phenomenon with a name.

It is up to you to decide what label to use but it should be as descriptive as possible so that when you see it or speak about it, you and other people will know exactly what is being described. There are many labels you could use but let's try the following: Sexuality Stunted Incontinence (SSI) or Sex Inhibiting Incontinence (SII). For the benefit of this explanation, we will use the former as our new concept.

The next step is to look for propositions. Put simply, a proposition is two or more concepts joined together in some way. In your case you would take your new concept, SSI, and investigate it further. To do this you may ask the following questions: 'How does it happen?', 'Why does it happen?', 'When does it happen?', 'Where does it happen?', and 'Who does it happen to?' By answering these questions you are in the process of building a model or theory, because models and theories are simply a collection of propositions.

Other concepts that could be linked to SSI are age and gender. For instance, if, after a thorough investigation, you noted that SSI was related to the age of the patient, then you can join these two concepts together by a statement. The statement could be one of the following:

- There is a relationship between age and SSI.
- People aged over 65 years are more likely to have SSI.
- There is a positive relationship between SSI and women aged over 70 years.
- There is a strong relationship between SSI and men aged over 65 years

These are only four examples of statements between concepts. Such statements are called propositions. The first one simply states that there is some relationship between age and SSI – it does not say what it is. The second proposition is much stronger and indicates a causal relationship between SSI and age. The third and fourth propositions bring in another concept – that of gender, so there are three concepts linked in these propositions.

You could identify other concepts that may be related to SSI, such as clinical setting, marital status, education, diagnoses, and time of day and create other propositions. What you have at the end of this is a theory or model.

When you hear researchers saying that they are going to test a theory or research a theory they are not really going to do that. What they will do is test the propositions to see if they are supported or refuted.

Let's say, you did test some of these propositions and found that men over the age of 65 who had urinary incontinence tended to also have problems expressing their sexuality or establishing or maintaining a normal sexual relationship. What you could do is write up these results. This might stimulate nurse researchers in other countries to see if they would get the same result. If they do, this could lay the foundations of evidence for practice so that when nurses assess men who have urinary incontinence and are age 65 they also assess their ability to express their sexuality. It could also influence other researchers to find a solution to the problem through physical or psychological means.

Congratulations, you are now a theorist and you have come up with a new SSI theory. To recap on how you did it – in your everyday practice you noticed something interesting which we will call a phenomenon. It appears that other nurses have noticed this too but there is nothing written about it in books or journals. You put a label onto it, called a concept, and begin to ask how, when, what, who and why questions. From these questions you identify other concepts that appear to be linked in some way with your concept. These links are propositions and, taken together, they provide you with a theory or model.

Now, to remain relevant, the propositional relationships within a theory need to be continually tested. If they hold up under continual testing over time you could say that the theory is valid. But, after several testings, it may be that the proposition fails. It is a bit like coming up with a recipe for a special cake. To get it just perfect, the ingredients must be correct, the baking must be correct, the oven must be pre-heated to an exact temperature and the cooking time must be precise. These are all concepts and when you put them together in a particular way, you have a perfect cake. You might make this cake 10 times without a problem but on the 11th time it fails to rise. In theory terms, it failed. So like a cake, your SSI theory can sometimes fail for a variety of reasons. The failure might be a one off or the theory may no longer be valid.

In *Figure 1.1* D-E is a one-way proposition whereas A-B-C are two way propositions. However, you will note that the concept D is not linked directly to the concepts F and G but indirectly through E.

Most of the other theorists covered in this book started their work in a similar way. They noticed phenomena such as people being in need of self-care (Orem, 1995), people needing to adapt to different situations they find

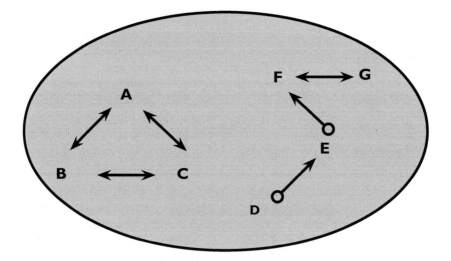

Figure 1.1. A diagrammatic representation of a nursing model or theory.

themselves in (Roy, 2003), or people needing to be independent in activities of daily living (Roper et al, 2000). You will note that these models/theories are composed of concepts and propositional links. For the models described in this book, the prior propositions have to some extent been tested through research and as a result the theory has been modified, supported or strengthened.

Types of theories

According to the sociologist, Merton (1968), there are three main types of theories: grand theories, mid-range theories and narrow range theories.

Grand theories

As their name suggests, grand theories are broad and highly abstract. They seek to describe and explain issues as broad as religion, medicine and nursing. For instance, it could be argued that Catholicism is a grand theory and seeks to describe and explain religion; that the biomedical theory seeks to describe and explain medicine; and that Orem's theory (1995) seeks to describe and explain nursing. In other words these three grand theories have for generations or centuries expressed what the phenomena of these disciplines are, and each has its own followers. As you would expect there are competing grand theories for religion, such as Calvinism or Judaism; for medicine, such as the psychological theory or sociological theory; and for nursing, such as Roy (2003) and Neuman (1995).

Grand theories take a global view of nursing and can act as an overriding philosophy for practice within a clinical setting. For instance, Orem's grand theory, as applied to a busy clinical setting, means that nursing within that setting is conceptualised and organised around the principle of self-care. If Roper et al's (2000) grand theory was used, the emphasis would be on helping patients address problems with their activities of daily living. This broad brush approach to theorising is useful as a guide for nurses' actions, beliefs, values and attitudes but they are not always helpful in identifying interventions for specific clinical problems. This is where mid-range theories help.

Mid-range theories

Mid-range theories are probably of greater benefit to practising nurses than the broader philosophical grand theories. This is because they are more precise, specific and focused and are normally based on the results of research. Therefore, they underpin evidence-informed practice. It is possible to create a mid-range theory from practice in a similar way to what we did above with the SSI theory. However, many research studies produce mid-range theories. Examples include the uncertainty in illness theory (Mishel, 1990), caring in perinatal nursing theory (Swanson, 1991), respite care theory (Nolan and Grant, 1992), maternal role attachment theory (Mercer, 1995), and comfort theory (Kolcaba, 2001). If you examine these mid-range theories carefully you will note that each of them is also composed of concepts linked by propositional statements. There do however tend to be fewer propositions in mid-range theories compared to grand theories. Here too, the testing of propositions through further research will check if the theory stands up to scrutiny.

It is also possible to get mid-range theories from researching the propositional links within grand theories. For example, Orem's self-care theory belongs in the category of grand theory. As mentioned above, it is composed of concepts ('self-care deficit', 'self-care agent', etc) and these concepts are linked to each other through propositional statements. By researching these propositions it is possible to come up with a mid-range theory such as a self-care deficit theory.

Narrow-range theories

Narrow-range theories are sometimes referred to as practice theories (McKenna and Slevin, 2008). They are much more specific and concrete than their grand or mid-range counterparts. These theories tell the nurse if a particular action will have a beneficial effect on a patient or if stopping another action will have a beneficial effect. You can see how these would be very useful as specific guides to practice. Examples that have become common practice include turning a patient two hourly to avoid the formation of pressure sores, visiting a patient pre-operatively so as to lessen the anxiety they experience post-operatively, and involving parents in the care of young hospitalised children to ensure good psychological recovery. Most practice theories are based on research and some are based on years of experience of what works and what does not work.

Model or theory: What is the difference?

What is the difference between theories and models? There has been much debate over this question in the literature but for the purposes of this book we take the view that there is no difference between a grand theory and a conceptual model. (Although we acknowledge and recognise that not all nurse theorists would agree with this position.).Think about it; a conceptual model is a framework composed of interrelated concepts. This also describes a grand theory. Let's take the explanation of a model a little further.

Think of a doll's house. In many regards it is a model or a representation of a real house. There may be rooms, toy furniture and toy dolls in it (e.g. concepts). It gives the child an indication of what the real thing is like and he or she can test out various ideas regarding where furniture is placed or how rooms can be decorated. A model of nursing (or grand theory) provides a representation of a way of viewing nursing. Like rearranging furniture, the nurse can see how different concepts work together.

In 1994 McKenna wrote that a nursing model is 'a representation of nursing that is systematically constructed and that assists practitioners in organising their thinking about what they do, and in the transfer of their thinking into practice for the benefit of patients and the profession'.

When Watson and Crick discovered DNA, they wanted to construct a simplified representative model of it so that they could show off their new discovery and explain it to the world. Therefore, on their lab bench they built the now famous double helix model out of an assortment of clamps and tubes. This simplified structure was also pleasing to look at and it helped explain DNA to the uninitiated. Similarly, Harry Beck's well-known map of the London Underground is a simplified model of a highly complex underground railway system. Armed with this one page map, millions of people each day traverse one of the largest cities in the world. Therefore, like the doll's house, or the underground map, a nursing model can be used to describe and explain complex phenomena in a simple way. However, many nurses perceive nursing models as doing the opposite; a common criticism of models being that they over-complicate nursing practice. This and other perceived limitations will be returned to in *Chapter 3*.

Does it matter which term we use?

It is interesting that many nurse scholars chose to use the term model rather than theory. This may be because nurse theorists were unsure of their ground and felt it would be too ambitious to call their early conceptualisations theories. There is some evidence for this. In their early writings nurse theorists such as Imogen King and Jean Watson referred to their work as models or conceptual frameworks. However, as the years went by, in later editions of their books or in their new texts they began to refer to their work as theories. For example, in her 1968 publication, King outlined her 'conceptual frame of reference' while in her 1971 book, she appeared to be heading 'towards a theory of nursing', which, when revised in 1981, revealed her 'theory of nursing'. This theoretical momentum is also evident in Watson's writings (Watson, 1979, 1985). Metatheorists disagree over the designations theory and model. For instance, Jacqueline Fawcett (2005) is convinced that nursing models are different from nursing theories. In contrast

Afaf Meleis (2007) argued that conceptualisations in nursing are all theories but only in a different stage of development. However, for the rest of this text, when we refer to a nursing model we will be referring simultaneously to a nursing grand theory.

Models and mid-range theories

The relationship between models and mid-range theories is the same as that between grand theories and mid-range theories. Models are broad and abstract representations of nursing and mid-range theories are narrower, more focused and research-driven representations of nursing. As alluded to above mid-range theories can be deduced from models by research being carried out on the relationships between different concepts within the model.

One- to three-dimensional models

Readers will notice that nursing models such as that of Orem, Roy, or Neuman are different to a doll's house or the London underground map. They all seek to simplify and be a representation of reality. However, a doll's house is three-dimensional because it has breadth, width and depth. In contrast, the map of the London underground is two-dimensional because it has only width and breadth. Nursing models are mostly one-dimensional in that they can be explained. However, most can also be represented in a two-dimensional diagram. Like a map the diagram of a nursing model can point staff members in a particular direction and show them important processes and structures in the clinical setting within which they find themselves.

To take this analogy a step further, different maps are needed for different purposes. If we wanted a map of London bus routes, sewer system or roadways, we would not consult the underground map. In nursing too we have different maps that seek to describe and explain nursing from different perspectives. At last count, there were over 50 grand theories of nursing and many more that are mid or narrow range. These can be seen simply as different maps to help us get around a very complex clinical landscape. In the following chapters some of these maps will be presented. Each has its strengths and weaknesses and each seeks to describe, explain and in some cases, prescribe nursing.

Why do we need models of nursing?

In *Chapter 3* we outline the limitations of nursing models and their usage. Here, we wish to provide an overview of their actual and potential benefits.

As a framework for the process of nursing

Over a number of years nurses have been taught to assess patients' problems, and plan, implement and evaluate their interventions. However, they have not been taught what to assess, how to plan, what to implement and how to evaluate. At their best, nursing models provide a theoretical template for the nursing process. For instance, you will see in *Chapter 5* how nurses can use Roy's model of adaptation to frame the nursing process. Through using Roy's model, nurses will know that they must assess how the patient is adapting in the four adaptation modes and identify what external and internal stimuli are impinging upon the patient's ability to adapt. The nursing care plan is focused on addressing these stimuli and returning the patient to the optimum level of adaptation. Without a nursing model, the nursing process is an empty approach to care. Therefore, to have meaning for practitioners the nursing process as a problem solving approach must be framed within a nursing model.

As a framework for research

As alluded to above, nursing models are composed of concepts linked by propositional statements. Each of these propositions can be turned into a research question or a hypothesis that can be tested by research. For instance, 'maintaining a safe environment' and 'mobilising' are two concepts within Roper et al's (2000) nursing model. These two concepts are linked by a simple propositional statement that there is a relationship between them. A research study could be undertaken to determine if those patients who have trouble mobilising also have more recorded accidents than those who do not. The results of this study could have beneficial effects on practice and contribute to the evidence that underpins practice.

As a framework for education

By definition, models of nursing attempt to identify what nursing is, who the recipients of nursing care are and what skills and knowledge practitioners should possess. It comes as no surprise that they can add good theoretical structure to a nursing curriculum. Furthermore, if the model that underpins the curriculum is the same one that is used in practice then the perennial theory–practice gap can be narrowed.

Patricia Benner in her novice-to-expert research (1984) indicated that, unlike expert practitioners, novices like strict guidelines within which to work. This explains why student nurses embrace structures like the nursing process and models of nursing and why experienced nurses find difficulty with them. McKenna and Slevin (2008) suggested that this is because expert nurses have their own implicit personal model of nursing based on years of experience. They find it difficult to replace this with a more formalised nursing model. It is also possible that this may be because experienced nurses have been used to working within the medical model (see *Chapter 2*).

Quality of care

As we approach the second decade of the 21st century, the provision of quality and safe care is central to nursing policy and practice worldwide. When care is founded on a systematic knowledge base it is more likely to be of a high standard. All nursing models stress the importance of planning and delivering high quality care. Furthermore, the evaluation of care quality is increasingly related to cost-effectiveness and clinical governance. For instance, using the models of Roper et al or Orem to underpin care help to reduce patient dependency and increase independence and autonomy. They also encourage the early detection of patients' problems and the cessation of non-nursing tasks.

Professionalisation

It has been argued that one hallmark of a profession is having a body of knowledge pertaining to its craft. Nursing models contribute to this body of knowledge by describing and explaining what nursing is. In addition, the development and use of models as a basis for practice is another characteristic of a profession. It was shown above that nursing models grow out of the phenomena that are central to nursing. Because of this, nursing models differentiate nursing from other disciplines. Not only can this show nurses themselves that they have a unique knowledge base but it can also illustrate that uniqueness to those from other disciplines and professions.

Summary

This chapter showed that theories are composed of concepts and the statements that link them. It pointed out that there were three types of theories in nursing: grand theories, mid-range theories and narrow-range or practice theories. Grand theories are synonymous with conceptual models. They tend to be abstract perspectives on nursing that can help practitioners assess, plan, implement and evaluate care. Not only can these models have a positive effect on the quality of nursing practice, they can also underpin quality education and research. Furthermore they are a welcome substitute to the archaic medical model and as such can influence the professionalisation of nursing.

References

Benner P (1984) *From Novice to Expert, Excellence and Power in Clinical Nursing Practice.* Addison-Wesley, Menlo Park, CA

Fawcett J (2005) *Contemporary Nursing Knowledge: Analysis and Evaluation of Nursing Models and Theories.* 2nd edn. FA Davis Company, Philadelphia

Kolcaba K (2001) Evolution of the mid range theory of comfort for outcomes research. *Nursing Outlook* **49**(2): 86–92

King I (1968) A conceptual frame of reference for nursing. *Nursing Research* **17**(1): 27–31

King I (1971) *Towards a Theory of Nursing.* John Wiley & Sons, New York

King I (1981) *A Theory of Nursing: Systems, Concepts, Process.* John Wiley & Sons, New York

McKenna HP (1994) *Nursing Theories and Quality of Care.* Avebury Press, Aldershot

McKenna HP, Slevin OD (2008) *Nursing Models, Theories and Practice.* Blackwell, Oxford

Meleis AI (2007) *Theoretical Nursing: Development and Progress.* 4th edn. Lippincott Williams and Wilkins, Philadelphia

Mercer RT (1995) *Becoming a Mother: Research from Rubin to the Present.* Springer Publishers, New York

Merton RK (1968) *Social Theory and Social Structure.* Free Press, New York

Mishel MH (1990) Reconceptualisation of the uncertainty in illness theory. *Image: The Journal of Nurse Scholarship* **22**: 256–61

Neuman B (1995) *The Neuman Systems Model.* 3rd edn. Appleton and Lange, Norwalk

Nolan M, Grant G (1992) Mid-range theory building and the nursing theory–practice gap: A respite care case study. *Journal of Advanced Nursing* **17**: 217–23

Orem DE (1995) *Nursing: Concepts of Practice.* 5th edn. McGraw Hill, New York

Roper N, Logan W, Tierney A (2000) *The Roper, Logan and Tierney Model of Nursing Based on Activities of Living.* Churchill Livingstone, Edinburgh

Roy C (2003) Reflections on nursing research and the Roy adaptation model. *Igaju-syoin Japanese Journal* **36**(1): 7–11

Swanson KM (1991) Empirical development of a mid-range theory of caring. *Nursing Research* **40**: 241–67

Watson J (1979) *A Model of Caring: An Alternative Health Care Model for Nursing Practice and Research.* New York, American Nurses Association. (Pub No. NP-59 3M 8179190)

Watson J (1985) *Nursing: Human Science and Care.* Appleton Century Crofts, New York

CHAPTER 2

Paradigms and metaparadigms

Most people do not like change. They feel comfortable with the status quo. Change can be confusing and anxiety provoking. This may be why individuals and groups do not often deviate from their usual habits. This lack of deviation may be caused by our desire for certainty. When we are not certain about something we are often ill at ease. Perhaps this explains why changes in clinical practice are often difficult to introduce.

The same applies to the nursing models we use to deliver care. In Chapter 1 we outlined that nursing models describe and explain what nursing is and how we should practice. For instance, Roper et al (2000) inform us that nursing is really about identifying problems with how patients are undertaking their activities of daily living. They direct us to help the patient become independent in undertaking these activities or cope with a lack of independence.

We have brought attention to the fact that currently there are over 50 different models of nursing and that these are like different road maps that we can follow. Most clinical nurses are familiar with only a small number of these and to change to another brings uncertainty and discomfort. The following sections will introduce you to how different nursing models are categorised and what is common among all of them.

This plethora of different models to guide our thinking and practice is not unique to nursing. In psychology there are many different models that seek to explain people's behaviour. These include psychoanalysis (Freud, 1949) and behaviourism (Skinner, 1938). Similarly, in sociology a range of different models have been formulated to describe and explain the family. These include nuclear and an extended models of the family unit (Williams et al, 2005).

The theoretical basis for nursing models

In essence, regardless of discipline, all models have their roots in a theory or group of theories. Nursing models are no exception. Their theoretical foundations have been identified as 'systems' theory, 'interactional' theory and 'developmental' theory. Some models also have a large behavioural component and hence the 'behavioural' theory is sometimes included as an additional category (McKenna, 1997)

Systems models

Systems models are largely based upon the general systems theory as put forward by Von Bertalanffy (1951). A 'system' is simply a collection of parts that interrelate as a whole entity for a particular purpose. A system has inputs, throughputs and outputs. If the system can affect and in turn be affected by, outside influences it is called an 'open system'. For instance, a clinical setting is an open system. There are inputs such as resources, staff and patients; there are throughputs, which are processes that take place in the setting; and there are outputs, such as patients being discharged and staff moving to other settings. In systems theory, all systems are part of larger suprasystems just as clinical settings are part of a hospital. This systems theory underpinned the nursing models constructed by Dorothy Johnson (1959), Calista Roy (1970), Betty Neuman (Neuman and Young, 1972), Rosemary Parse (1981) and Joyce Fitzpatrick (1982).

Interactional models

Interactional nursing models are seen as having their basis in symbolic interactionist theory (Blumer, 1969). This theory emphasises the relationships between people and the roles they play in society. Nursing is seen as a social activity, an interactional process between the nurse and the patient.

The interactional models of nursing were conceived in the 1950s and early 1960s and the most renowned are those of Hildegard Peplau (1952), Joyce Travelbee (1966), Ida Orlando (1961), and Imogene King (1968). These models tend to view nursing as an interactional process that is concerned with the development of a therapeutic interpersonal relationship between patients and nurses. Peplau (1987) defined nursing as a therapeutic interpersonal process while Travelbee (1966) asserted that nursing is an interpersonal process between two human beings, one of whom needs assistance because of an illness and the other who is able to give such assistance. Orlando (1961) emphasised that the nurse–patient relationship should be based on planned action. King's theory (1968) focused on nursing as a process of human interaction between the nurse and patient whereby each perceives the other in the situation and, through communication, they set goals and explore and agree on the means to achieve goals.

Developmental models

Developmental nursing models take their origins from the work of Freud (1949). The central themes are growth, development, maturation and change. Within developmental theory it is argued that from the moment of conception to the moment of death, human beings are constantly developing. This maturation may be social, physiological, psychological or spiritual. Development is seen as an ongoing process in which individuals must pass through various stages and, with each transition, they achieve greater self-responsibility. Nursing involves removing or preventing barriers to this natural developmental process. We can include among the 'developmental models' the work of Margaret Newman (1979).

Behavioural models

These nursing models owe much to the work of Abraham Maslow (1954) and his theory relating to the hierarchy of needs and motivation. Because of this, they are often called 'human needs models' (Meleis, 2007). These nursing models assume that individuals normally function in society by their own efforts, that is, they meet their needs, carry out their activities of living and undertake their self-care requirements. In most cases we do not need others to do this for us. Therefore, independence in basic human needs is the focus for nursing action within 'behavioural models'. This category includes the work of Virginia Henderson (1966), Dorothea Orem (1995), Martha Rogers (1980), and Nancy Roper et al (2000).

Philosophically two main methods for the development of nursing models have been identified: the inductive approach and the deductive approach (McKenna and Slevin, 2008). The inductive method suggests that theory is developed from the observation of practice or from the personal experience of the theorist. In Chapter 1 we outlined how nurses can notice phenomena in practice and from giving these phenomena their attention they can identify concepts, propositions and then models. In this case the nurse is reasoning from the 'specific' situation to 'general' situations.

In contrast the deductive approach leads to the development of nursing models from existing theories such as those outlined above. We have seen how nursing models can develop from systems, interactional, developmental and behavioural theories. Here the theorist is reasoning from the 'general' theory to the 'specific' model.

Although some nursing theorists maintain that they have derived their models from observing practice (Roy, 1980; Orem, 1995), most take as their starting point one or more of those broad theories outlined above. Therefore, in nursing science a mixture of induction and deduction has been used to develop models of practice. It could of course be argued that developing a model inductively from simply observing practice is not very scientific and the model would have to go through rigorous testing before it is validated. An alternative argument is that if nursing models are deduced from the existing theories of other disciplines they may have difficulty explaining the actuality of nursing practice. This failure of models to reflect reality and the implications this has for the 'real–ideal gap' will be explored in the next section.

The theory–practice gap

Over the years several research studies have highlighted the existence of a 'theory–practice gap' (Bendall, 1975; Nolan, 1989; Maben et al, 2006) This commonly refers to the dichotomy that exists between what students are taught in class and what they experience in clinical practice. However, the divide between theory and practice does not just affect nursing students. It may be apparent to qualified staff that their methods of assessing, planning, implementing and evaluating care bear little resemblance to what the journal articles or textbooks suggest. This may cause them to experience cognitive dissonance. Festinger (1964) used this term to explain the anxiety experienced by those whose behaviour is inconsistent with their values. If nurses adopt a specific nursing model as part of their value system, then they may experience cognitive dissonance when they find that these values are inconsistent with what they practise.

But what effect do nursing models have on the theory–practice gap? There is consensus in the literature that models should emerge from practice and return to practice (McKenna and Slevin, 2008). However, in reality models of nursing invariably come from an academic background and most theorists have been away from practice and the reality of nursing for many years. Therefore, since most models are not being formulated by practising nurses, this encourages the theory–practice gap to remain. In taking a broader view Meleis (2007: 50) felt that: 'Nurse theorists were developing theories in isolation, researchers pursued questions of interest only to educators and administrators and practitioners pursued their practices whilst oblivious to what the other two groups were doing.'

There are other possible reasons why nursing models may lead to a widening of the theory–practice gap. They include the American origin of various nursing models and the jargon used by nurse theorists to structure their models. Much of the division stems from nurse practitioners seeing themselves as 'doers' and the theorists as 'thinkers'.

It is not clear whether nurses would still hold these opinions if they had a better understanding of the models in question. After all, many nurses have not been given the time, the opportunity, the support or the education to comprehend them or implement them properly. Furthermore, the perceived contribution of nursing models to the theory–practice gap may have been less if they had not been introduced by nurse management using a 'power-coercive' approach (McKenna, 1997).

Notwithstanding these views it can also be argued that it is only by using nursing models that theory and practice may eventually meet. One such approach is for educators to underpin curricula with nursing models that match practice. If a nursing curriculum is structured around a particular nursing model and the same model is used by practitioners then the theory–practice gap could be bridged for both students and staff.

However, nursing models may become outmoded and no longer reflect the reality of nursing. For instance, unless they have undergone revisions, amendments and updating, we could argue that nursing models developed over half a century ago, like those of Peplau (1952) and Roy (1971) have limited currency in the 21st century. How then do those models change and how does nursing knowledge renew itself?

Knowledge development in nursing: Revolution, evolution or convolution?

The Oxford English Dictionary (1981: 126) defined paradigm as 'a pattern or model, or an exemplar'. Therefore, paradigms are simply another word for models. The person best known for his work on paradigms is Thomas Kuhn. In 1970 he wrote a book called *The Structure of Scientific Revolution*. Put simply, Kuhn postulated that society adopted a particular paradigm to explain how things worked. This paradigm may be the favoured perspective for many years. He called this period 'normal science'. However, at some stage the paradigm is no longer able to explain a new phenomenon and so a revolution occurs and there is a search for a new paradigm among several competing ones. Eventually another one is adopted and this leads to another period of normal science until the next paradigm shift is required.

There are many examples of paradigm shifts in the history of the world. In Chapter 1 we highlighted how at one time 'normal science' believed that the earth was the centre of the universe. However, this paradigm became obsolete when Galileo used his telescope to prove that Copernicus was correct in his belief that the earth revolved around the sun. Here, a revolution in beliefs occurred and there was a shift to a new paradigm. Other paradigm shifts include a shift from a belief that the earth was flat to the earth being a sphere, and a shift from Newton's theory of gravity to Einstein's theory of relativity. Paradigm shifts occurred because the old paradigms were not able to explain new experiences or solve new problems.

Therefore, Thomas Kuhn believed that new knowledge and understanding was the result of a series of revolutions (see *Figure 2.1*). Often these revolutions lead to a completely different way of viewing and explaining things. This has attractions for nurses because, with new health technologies, they often have to change dramatically their knowledge or skills base. For instance the recent shift from hospital-focused care to community-focused care has placed new challenges on community nursing. We could include here too the shift in nurse education provision from hospital-based colleges of nursing to university schools of nursing.

In contrast to Kuhn's paradigm shifts, a philosopher and epidemiologist called Larry Laudan (1977) came up with a different explanation for how knowledge develops (see *Figure 2.2*). Laudan believed that new knowledge evolved from previous knowledge. Put simply, new knowledge builds on older knowledge and rather than there being a paradigm shift there is a paradigm stretch. This means that the paradigm evolves rather than changes. Laudan's evolutionary approach to knowing is an attractive one for nurses

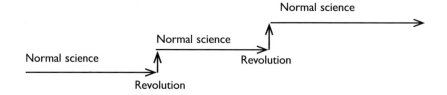

Figure 2.1.A depiction of Kuhn's revolutionary paradigm shifts.

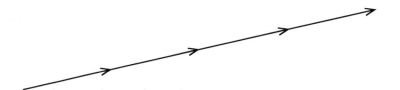

Figure 2.2. Larry Laudan evolutionary approach to knowledge development.

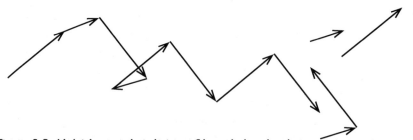

Figure 2.3. Meleis's convoluted view of knowledge development in nursing.

because it recognises that nursing's knowledge base is growing steadily and that we as a profession are continually evolving.

But do these two views of knowledge development really explain what is happening in nursing? Afaf Meleis (2007), the Egyptian born metatheorist, argued that the revolutionary and evolutionary approaches to knowledge development are too simplistic on their own to explain nursing's experience. She used the term 'convolution' to explain how nursing knowledge has developed (see *Figure 2.3*). To Meleis, nursing as a discipline has progressed not through evolution or revolution but through a convolution of peaks, troughs, detours, backward steps and crises. There may be some truth in this as nursing is still a young scientific discipline and often knowledge development is confusing and uncoordinated. Why else would there be so many different models of nursing all claiming to be correct? It may be that we are currently placed in what Kuhn (1977) called a pre-paradigmatic stage of development. In other words we have not really decided on which paradigm best explains what nursing is and what it does.

Metaparadigm: The 'essential elements' of nursing models

Regardless of how nursing models are categorised, there is agreement in the literature that each one must include views on four essential elements. The origin for this view comes from a seminal study undertaken in 1974 by Torres and Yura. They surveyed a sample of 50 American baccalaureate nursing programmes accredited by the National League of Nursing. They concluded that the elements of nursing, health, man and society were central to all the programmes reviewed. These concepts have more recently been refined as; nursing, health, the person and the environment. When referring to these elements Jacqueline Fawcett (1989) used the term 'metaparadigm'.

Fawcett (1989: 67) defined a 'metaparadigm' as: 'The global perspective of any discipline that acts as an encapsulating structure within which conceptual frameworks develop.'

Therefore, a metaparadigm is another word for a 'world view'. Most professions have a single metaparadigm from which many models emerge. For example, the concepts of design, material, shape and creation would make up the metaparadigm of architecture and from this many different architectural models have developed. Similarly, the metaparadigm of medicine is composed of concepts such as patients, diagnoses and therapeutics.

During the 1970s and 1980s nursing authors wrote extensively about the importance of the metaparadigm of nursing, health, the person and the environment for the advancement of nursing practice and nursing science

(Fawcett, 2005; Meleis, 2007). The argument was put forward that unless a conceptual framework includes assumptions about these four elements it cannot be considered to be a nursing model. This makes sense since how could there be a model of nursing that did not refer to nursing or to health or to the person or to the environment where care took place.

We would wish to stress the interdependence of these essential elements and the need for fluidity and interconnections between them. However, as you would expect it is easy to be critical of the metaparadigm. One criticism is that having nursing as one of the essential elements leads to a tautology. A tautology is where there is repetition of meaning or where different words are used to say the same thing twice. In other words, how can nursing be one of the essential elements of nursing. Another criticism is that if you remove nursing from the metaparadigm, what is left (person, health environment) could relate to medicine, any other health profession or even the discipline of health and safety. Stevens (1979) excluded environment, while Kim (1983) excluded health. However, most authors support the metaparadigm in its entirety.

Afaf Meleis (2007) uses the term 'domain' rather than metaparadigm. Although it does not have the exact same components as the metaparadigm, it has a similar meaning. She defined domain (2007: 112) as 'the perspective and territory of a discipline.' She goes further than Fawcett and identifies seven concepts as central to the domain of nursing. These are: nursing client, transitions, interaction, nursing process, environment, nursing therapeutics, and health.

To illustrate the relationship between these concepts: Meleis (2007) believes that the nurse interacts (interaction) with a human being in a health/illness situation (nursing client) who is an integral part of his sociocultural context (environment) and who is in some sort of transition or is anticipating a transition (transition); the nurse-patient interactions are organised around some purpose (nursing process), and the nurse uses some actions (nursing therapeutics) to enhance, bring about or facilitate health (health).

Fawcett (2006) ably addresses the criticisms levelled at her perception of the metaparadigm. She also appears to be coming closer to the ideas of Meleis in that she specifies that 'nursing' within her four-component metaparadigm does include nursing therapeutics, and 'person' does include groups and communities. Therefore when trying to encapsulate what is the 'world view' of nursing, it is legitimate to use either metaparadigm or domain. For this text we will use metaparadigm.

Although each nursing model deals with the four essential elements of the metaparadigm, they may stress different aspects and see them in different relations to one another (See *Figure 2.4*). Therefore, how nursing, health, person and environment are described and defined vary greatly from nursing model to nursing model. It could be argued that such a diversity of views on the same concepts only serves to enrich nursing as a discipline.

Health

Within nursing models, health has been represented as a level of adaptation (King, 1968; Roy, 1980), an appropriate level of independence (Peplau, 1952; Roper et al, 2000), a state of wholeness (Rogers, 1980; Orem, 1995), or a desired value (Johnson, 1959; Travelbee, 1966). Neuman and Young (1972) discussed health as 'wellness', while Orlando (1961) outlined the importance of 'mental and physical comfort'.

Nursing

Among nursing scholars, there is still no generally accepted definition of 'nursing'. This may be because nursing is a complicated discipline with many complex phenomena. Such complexity is reflected in how nursing is explicated within nursing models.

Some nursing models view nursing as 'assisting as necessary' (Orem, 1995; Roper et al, 2000). Those models that have their focus on psychiatric care tend to envisage 'nursing' as an 'interpersonal process' (Peplau, 1952; Orlando, 1961; Travelbee, 1966). King (1968) is a firm advocate of interactional theory, believing that nursing is really all about 'social interaction'.

Other descriptions of nursing include, 'supporting the patients' adaptation' (Roy, 1970; Rogers, 1980), 'helping patient achieve equilibrium' (Johnson, 1959), 'participating with the patient's health experiences' (Parse, 1987), 'assisting persons to utilise their own resources' (Newman, 1979) and 'intervening at primary, secondary and tertiary levels of prevention' (Neuman and Young, 1972).

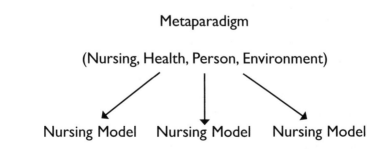

Metaparadigm

(Nursing, Health, Person, Environment)

Nursing Model   Nursing Model   Nursing Model

Figure 2.4. The relationship between the metaparadigm and nursing models.

Person

Over the years nursing's view of the person has changed from the Cartesian anatomical and physiological entity with mind–body dichotomy, to being an individual with biological, spiritual, emotional, social and cognitive dimensions. This 'holistic' image tends to permeate most nursing models.

Many nursing models perceive the person as 'someone who has differing and changing needs' (Henderson, 1966; Roper et al, 2000). Orem (1995) focused on the person as a self-care agent; Parse (1987), Neuman and Young (1972), King (1968) and Johnson (1959) saw the person as an 'open system', while Rogers (1980) and Newman (1979) describe him/her as an 'energy field'. Several other descriptions exist. For example an 'adapter to stress' (Roy, 1970), a 'behaving human organism' (Orlando, 1961), or simply an 'evolving irreplaceable individual' (Travelbee, 1966). More recently, the view of person has been expanded to include families and communities (McKenna and Slevin, 2008)

The environment

Nursing models tend to view the environment as not just what is external to the person, but also what is internal (Roy, 1980; Orem, 1995; Neuman and Young, 1972). Other models portray the environment as the 'arena where the person functions', or 'where he/she gets sustenance' (Orlando, 1961; Travelbee, 1966).

Newman (1979) and Rogers (1980) considered the environment to be an 'energy field' that is part of the 'life process'. King (1968), in keeping with her views on the 'person', believed the environment to be an 'open system' in interaction with human beings. Corresponding with her assumptions regarding interpersonal relationships, Peplau (1952) described the environment as 'microcosms of significant others with whom the person interacts'.

From the above descriptions it can be seen that, although all nursing models deal with the metaparadigm, they tend to view its essential elements from different perspectives. There are, of course, some commonalities and one can see the influences of the underlying systems, and interactional, developmental and behavioural theories. Nevertheless the basic metaparadigm elements have been moulded to suit the different perspectives of the individual theorists and as such each model is uniquely different.

Summary

This chapter was entitled paradigms and metaparadigms. It highlighted that models are simply paradigms that can grow inductively from practice or deductively from other larger more established theories. The latter approach to the development of nursing models can perpetuate the continuation of the theory–practice gap. It was also stressed that on occasions there is a gap between existing knowledge and how new realities are explained and understood and that this gap may be bridged through revolution, evolution or convolution. Finally, the metaparadigm was described and its role in shaping nursing models explained.

References

Bendall E (1975) *So You Passed, Nurse*. Royal College of Nursing, London

Blumer H (1969) *Symbolic Interactionism: Perspective and Method*. Prentice Hall, Englewood Cliffs, New Jersey

Fawcett J (1989) *Analysis and Evaluation of Conceptual Models of Nursing*. FA Davis, Philadelphia

Fawcett J (2005) *Contemporary Nursing Knowledge: Analysis and Evaluation of Nursing Models and Theories* 2nd edn. FA Davis Company, Philadelphia

Fawcett J (2006) Personal communication

Festinger L (1964) *Conflict Decision and Dissonance*. Tavistock Publications, London

Fitzpatrick JJ (1982) Fitzpatrick's model. In Fitzpatrick JJ et al (Eds) *Nursing Models: Application to Psychiatric Mental Health Nursing*. Brady & Co, Maryland, USA

Freud S (1949) *An Outline of Psychoanalysis*. WW Norton, New York

Henderson V (1966) *The Nature of Nursing: A definition and Its Implications for Practice, Education and Research*. Collier Macmillan, London

Johnson DE (1959) The nature of a science of nursing. *Nursing Outlook* **7**: 291–4

Kim HS (1983) *The Nature of Theoretical Thinking in Nursing*. Norwalk, Conn, Appleton-Century-Crofts

King I (1968) A conceptual frame of reference for nursing. *Nursing Research* **17**(1): 27–31

Kuhn T (1970) *The Structure of Scientific Revolution* (2nd Edn). University of Chicago Press, Chicago

Kuhn TS (1977) *The Structure of Scientific Revolution* (3rd Edn). University of Chicago Press, Chicago

Laudan L (1977) *Progress and Its Problems: Towards a Theory of Scientific Growth*. University of California Press, Berkley

Levine ME (1966) Adaptation and assessment. A rationale for nursing intervention. *American Journal of Nursing* **66**(11): 2450–53

Maben J, Latter S, Macleod Clark J (2006) The theory–practice gap: Impact of professional-bureaucratic work conflict on newly-qualified nurses. *Journal of Advanced Nursing* **55**(4): 465–77

Maslow AH (1954) *Motivation and Personality*. Harper & Row, New York

McKenna HP (1997) *Nursing Models and Theories*. Routledge, London

McKenna HP, Slevin OD (2008) *Vital Notes for Nurses: Nursing Models, Theories and*

Practice. Blackwell, London

Meleis AI (2007) *Theoretical Nursing: Development and Progress*. 4th edn. Lippincott Williams and Wilkins, Philadelphia

Neuman B, Young RJ (1972) A model for teaching total person approach to patient problems. *Nursing Research* **21**(3): 264–9

Newman MA (1979) *Theory Development in Nursing*. FA Davis & Co, Philadelphia

Nolan PW (1989) *Psychiatric Nursing Past and Present: The Nurses' Viewpoint*. University of Bath, Unpublished PhD Thesis

Orem DE (1995) *Nursing: Concepts of Practice*. 5th edn. McGraw Hill, New York

Orlando I (1961) *The Dynamic Nurse–Patient Relationship. Function, Process, and Principles*. GP Putnam & Sons, New York

Oxford English Dictionary (1981) Oxford University Press, Oxford

Parse RR (1981) *Man-Living-Health: A Theory of Nursing*. John Wiley & Sons, New York

Parse RR (1987) *Nursing Science: Major Paradigms, Theories and Critiques*. WB Saunders, Philadelphia

Paterson JG, Zderak LT (1976) *Humanistic Nursing*. John Wiley & Sons, New York

Peplau HE (1952) *Interpersonal Relations in Nursing*. GP Putnam & Sons, New York

Peplau HE (1987) Nursing science: A historical perspective. In: Parse RR (ed) *Nursing Science: Major Paradigms, Theories and Critiques*. WB Saunders Co, Philadelphia

Rogers ME (1980) *An Introduction to a Theoretical Basis of Nursing*. 2nd edn. FA Davis & Co, Philadelphia

Roper N, Logan W, Tierney AJ (2000) *The Roper-Logan-Tierney Model of Nursing Based on Activities of Living*. Churchill-Livingstone, Edinburgh

Roy C (1970) Adaptation - a conceptual framework for nursing. *Nursing Outlook* **18**(3) 42–5

Roy C (1971) Adaptation - a basis for nursing practice. *Nursing Outlook* **19**(4) 254–7

Roy C (1980) The Roy adaptation model. In: Riehl JP, Roy C (eds) *Conceptual Models for Nursing Practice*. New York, Appleton-Century-Crofts

Skinner BF (1938) *The Behaviour of Organisms: An Experimental Analysis*. Appleton-Century-Crofts, New York,

Stevens BJ (1979) *Nursing Theory: Analysis, Application, Evaluation*. Little, Brown & Co, Boston

Torres G, Yura N (1974) *Today's Conceptual Framework: Its Relationship to the Curriculum Development Process*. Pub. No. 15-1529. New York, National League of Nursing

Travelbee J (1966) *Interpersonal Aspects of Nursing*. FA Davis, Philadelphia

Von Bertalanffy L (1951) General systems theory: A new approach to unity of science. *Human Biology* 121: 303–61

Watson J (1979) *A Model of Caring: An Alternative Health Care Model for Nursing Practice and Research*. American Nurses' Association, New York

Williams B, Sawyer SC, Wahlstrom CM (2005) *Marriages, Families & Intimate Relationships*. Pearson, Boston, MA

CHAPTER 3

The history of nursing models

Florence Nightingale has been recognised as the first nurse to attempt to theorise about her craft. Although she believed that the very elements of nursing were all but unknown, she expressed the firm view that nursing knowledge should be distinct from medical knowledge (Nightingale, 1859). Nightingale is therefore credited with laying the foundations for the first model of nursing.

That she favoured constructing a model to describe and explain nursing is not surprising. After all she had a love of mathematical models to the extent that she kept a statistical textbook under her pillow. When we examine her work, particularly her *Notes on Nursing* (1859), we can extract her views on what would be the modern day metaparadigm. Her view of nursing, person, health and environments was influenced greatly by her time in Kaiserwerth, Germany, Dublin, Ireland, Paris, France and in Constantinople, Turkey during the Crimean War.

In 1854, Nightingale was horrified by news reports in the *London Times* by the Crimean war correspondent William Howard Russell. Soldiers were dying from starvation and neglect rather than from the wounds of battle. Russell compared this to how the French Sisters of Mercy cared for the French soldiers and he asked whether there were like-minded women in England who would go to the Crimea and nurse the British soldier (Walshe, 1929). Nightingale, believed that she was a person who could do this and she lobbied influential politicians and, after getting permission, set sail for Constantinople with a group of 38 nurses and religious sisters. Their base was the notorious Barrack Hospital at Scutari, across the Bosporus from Constantinople. When she arrive there, she noticed that it was filthy, with wounded soldiers lying in muddy corridors with rats running rampant. She sent those who had accompanied her from England into the market of Constantinople to buy linen for bandages and she ordered the army to make wooden beds.

Although Nightingale (1859) stated that obedience was 'suitable praise for a horse' she did order her colleagues to follow the directions of the military physicians. This may have had more to do with her military and upper class background than with her belief that nurses were subservient to physicians. In fact she was of the opinion that medicine and nursing should be clearly differentiated from each other.

Between caring for the wounded and dying, she and the other women began the Herculean task of cleaning the Barrack Hospital. Some of the windows had not been open in years and in order to get fresh water a dead horse had to be removed from the drinking well. She noticed that fresh air and cleanliness seemed to make a difference. She believed in the miasmic view of disease that it is carried along in the atmosphere. Therefore, it is not surprising that Nightingale's model of nursing laid great emphasis on the importance of the right caring environment with cleanliness, fresh air and fresh water.

Nightingale believed that the role of nursing was to put patients in the best condition for nature to act upon them. Therefore, she did not accept that doctors cured; rather nature or a healthy environment was responsible for curing. At the end of *Notes on Nursing* (1859: 112) she argued:

> *It is said that medicine is a curative process. It is no such thing; medicine is the surgery of functions, as surgery is that of limbs and organs. Neither can do anything but remove obstructions; neither can cure; nature alone cures. Surgery removes the bullet out of the limb, which is the obstruction to cure, but nature heals the wound. So it is with medicine; the function of an organ becomes obstructed; medicine, as far as we know, assists nature to remove the obstruction, but does nothing more.*

When she returned to London she was unwell with what was termed Crimean fever. The people and the Government wanted to thank her for her work in the Crimea and they started the Nightingale Fund. With the proceeds from this she set about establishing the first School of Nursing at St Thomas's Hospital in London. This was not welcomed by British physicians who 'felt the training of nursing ought to be entirely in their hands and were very much afraid that if nurses were trained to take care of the sick, they would almost surely want to practise as physicians or as healers of some kind and the result would be a great addition to the number of quacks and charlatans' (Walshe, 1929: 233).

The curriculum at St Thomas's was based on what could loosely be called Nightingale's model of nursing. Inherent in this is the strong belief that since it is nature that cures, nurses may be in as good a position as physicians, if not better, to place the patient in the best position for nature to do its work. This also had the effect of distancing them from their previous subservient position to the physician. Nightingale (1859: 135) stated: 'if I have succeeded in any measure in … showing what true nursing is, and what it is not, my object will have been answered.' From St Thomas's nurses spread across the world to set up similar schools of nursing. They were not only vilified by doctors. Bellevue Hospital in New York requested and got three of St Thomas's graduates; on several occasions while going to and from their quarters they were met with a volley of stones from the older and old fashioned nurses who felt they were being displaced (Walshe, 1929).

While Nightingale and her nurses were pushing forward the frontiers of nursing practice, she also was leaving a legacy that may have been responsible for holding back advances in nursing for many subsequent years. Nightingale was a very religious woman and religion also permeated the nurse training programme she propagated. As alluded to above, she was also very involved with the military and in fact is just as famous in history for her army reforms as she was for her nursing reforms. This military and religious background formed the context for much of nursing for future generations. Until recently, religious terms such as sister and vocation, and military terms such as hierarchy, nursing officer, duty, and uniform brought with them the worst excesses of obedience in the nursing discipline.

Nightingale had two great loves of her life. These were politics and statistical research. It was unfortunate that her intense interest in these subjects was not passed on through her commitment to nurse training. In contrast, male medical students often excelled at these subjects. Furthermore, in the latter part of the 19th century physicians and nurses were also separated by their gender, social class, language and education.

Despite the efforts of Nightingale and her rapidly expanding systems of nurse training schools, there were still some untrained nurses who were 'Sairey Gamp' like figures (Dickens, 1866) In Martin Chuzzlewit, Dickens described nurse Gamp in the following way:

She is a nurse of sorts whose specialty lies in the polar extremities of life, the lying in and the laying out. The face of Mrs Gamp – the nose in particular – was somewhat red and swollen, and it was difficult to enjoy her society without becoming conscious of a smell of spirits.

Walshe (1929: 217) pointed out that in the mid-19th century nurses were:

menials with no character and the one thing that was hoped for from them was that they would keep sober. The younger ones among them, especially if attractive, were seduced and temptations of all kinds, liquor, graft, sex, were associated with their lives.

While this was referred to nurses more than 10 years after Nightingale returned from the Crimea, we can see from this popular depiction that nursing as an occupation was perceived as squalid, unscientific and unprofessional. In contrast, medicine was a university course populated mainly by middle class males from rich and privileged backgrounds.

In her long lifetime (1820–1910) nightingale was not the only nurse theorist to consider the what and why of nursing. Norris (1970) reminded us that in the late 19th and early 20th centuries there were some isolated instances of nurses attempting to conceptualise. He described Shaw's work in the 1880s on nurse–patient interaction, and public health nurses' early experimentation with self-care. However, these and other efforts were pre-empted by the adoption of the medical model that was to permeate nurse education and practice for most of the 20th century. It could be argued that the resultant theoretical hiatus in nurse theorising persisted until Peplau began to conceptualise psychiatric nursing in the 1950s.

The medical model

The medical model is a good model for medicine but not for nursing. It can be traced back to the ancient Greek teachings of Hippocrates, Aristotle and Galen. It is mainly focused on the physical body and at its most simplistic it views the body as a machine. The machine is made up of parts and systems and when a part breaks down it must be fixed. One way of fixing it is to provide some oral chemical agent, almost as oil for the internal cogs and wheels. Another way is to open the machine and remove the part, repair it or replace it. Many members of the public accept this model of medicine and even today new replacement parts and new chemical compounds are welcomed and widely lauded by the medical fraternity, the media and society.

The medical model emphasised that illness was caused by genetic, biochemical, traumatic or pathological disturbances and was mainly treated by medication or surgery. Social and psychological factors had little currency within this framework. This perspective of the body as a machine encouraged the adoption of a philosophy of reductionism where human beings were reduced to the level of anatomical parts and physiological systems. In contrast, nursing models take a more holistic approach and recognise that people have psychological, social and spiritual as well as physical dimensions. Nursing models take pride in stating that people are more than simply the sum of their parts.

Nursing and the medical model

The servile 'handmaiden' image of nursing can partly be due to Nightingale's emphasis on military and religious obedience. However, it can also be due to a tenacious reliance on the medical model. The medical model does not allow for independent nursing action and armed with this model the nurse is ill equipped to envisage and help the patient as a whole person.

In the early to mid-20th century, nursing education and management laid out a philosophy that the role of the nurse was to assist the doctor. If this was indeed the case, then it was important that they were well prepared for this role. Doctors were asked to teach nurses in the classroom and on the ward and many popular nursing textbooks were written by doctors (Walshe, 1929). Later, Peplau (1987) argued that those who teach, control the content of an occupation. Through such brainwashing, nurses inherited a slavish adherence to a Cartesian reductionist philosophy where human beings were little more than disease entities (McKenna, 1997).

Most physicians based their treatment philosophy on this fundamental tenet of reductionism. This implies that all behavioural phenomena must be conceptualised in terms of physiochemical principles. Over the years this basic precept has been accepted not only by many healthcare professionals but also by the public. Society has got used to the idea of a pill for every ill or the repair of internal damage through surgery. This reductionist view appears to ignore the many social and psychological influences to which individuals are susceptible. Under this model, the fact that a patient may be unemployed, have six children, or was worried about his sick wife was not a matter for great consideration by those who propounded the medical model. Traditional medical education focused on the physical sciences of biology, physics, chemistry, histology and pathology. It has only recently that the study of sociology, psychology and philosophy has been introduced to the medical curriculum.

Within the medical model the preliminary assessment is of great importance to physicians. The initial examination will ultimately lead to the recognition of signs and symptoms; these are categorised into patterns which in turn form the basis for diagnostic labelling. Such labelling has a dehumanising effect. Nurses also have slipped almost imperceptibly into using diagnostic labels to refer to patients – the schizophrenic in villa A or the coronary in bed C. In addition, when using the nursing process, nurses often tend to use the language of symptoms to describe client behaviours, and classify clients into diagnostic types.

As well as having a major input into teaching practices and curriculum design many questions in nursing examinations reflected the medical model. Similarly, nursing care studies published within professional nursing journals rarely escaped being tinged with this ideology. Their sub-headings tended to focus on aetiology, symptomatology, medical history, diagnostic tests and treatment strategies. The role of nursing in such care studies was obscure.

Within the medical model, knowing the diagnosis determines the treatment goals. These are seldom client-centred and the patient must willingly assume the sick role and agree to co-operate with treatment. Parsons (1952) recognised that clients, as exemplified by the sick role, have the right to be relieved from social roles and the right not to be held responsible for their illness or condition. They are however, obliged to seek professional help and to try their best to get well. You can see how this view of how to behave when sick has permeated society and most people behave in this way when faced with medical intervention.

As part of their education, nurses were discouraged from providing information to the patient about their illness and possible prognosis – this is the doctor's job. While the clinical camaraderie may present the facade of the egalitarian team approach, the doctor as the healer was viewed as superior to all other healthcare disciplines. Such a focus does not allow for independent action and a danger exists that it may lead practitioners to ignore aspects of the client which do not fit neatly within the boundaries of the medical model.

Our education preparation within the medical model fostered a fascination with cure, with care being placed in a secondary position. Like our medical colleagues, many nurses have shown preferences for work in busy acute settings where technology is respected and so called technical skills are given high status. The more sedate long-stay wards and care of the older adult units where care should be paramount are less popular choices among ambitious nurses and to this day tend to be staffed with large numbers of untrained personnel.

Although the medical approach to modern nursing is becoming increasingly queried, there is evidence that it still remains a major influence in the delivery of care. As a result of a worldwide shortage of doctors and legislation that reduces the number of hours they can work many medical duties are being transferred to nurses. In turn, nurses are transferring much of their 'basic nursing care' to untrained assistive personnel. The danger is obvious; will clinical nurses become 'mini doctors' and assistive personnel become 'maxi nurses' (McKenna et al, 2007)

It has to be accepted that the medical model has made a valued contribution to the health and wellbeing of the population. Advances in medically oriented cures have freed many clients from the effects of disturbing symptomatology and contributed to their early discharge and a healthier lifestyle. Therefore, it is important that nurses take cognisance of these factors and realise the imprudence of rejecting the medical model in its entirety. Within any nursing model/theory the biological and pathological perspective of the individual should be acknowledged.

Although the medical frame of reference is undergoing critical examination, a trace of traditional subordination to physicians and the carrying out of their orders, may remain with nursing for some time to come.

Meanwhile, nursing's disenchantment with the pervasiveness of the medical model was one of the main reasons for the rediscovery of nursing models.

The re-discovery of nursing models

The North American story

As can be seen in the previous section, Nightingale's early efforts to conceptualise nursing were eclipsed by the adoption of the medical model that was to permeate nurse education and practice for many years. The resultant theoretical hiatus in nursing persisted until the mid-20th century. The following reasons have been put forward to explain why renewed attempts at conceptualising nursing should have occurred in America in the 1950s:

- Disenchantment with the medical model.
- The wartime employment and liberation of women.
- The arrival of university education for nurses.
- The establishment in 1952 of *Nursing Research*, the world's first academic nursing journal.
- The quest for professional status.
- The need to develop a scientific basis for nursing.
- The increased expectations and involvement of the patient.

Psychiatric nursing took the lead in the reappearance of theoretical thinking among nurses. Hildegard Peplau, a psychiatric nurse, is credited with formulating the first contemporary conceptual model for nursing. Her work (Peplau, 1952)not only influenced, but also formed the basis for, later attempts to develop further nursing models. The most notable among these theorists were Virginia Henderson (Henderson and Harmer, 1955), Dorothea Orem (1959), Dorothy Johnson (1959) and Lydia Hall (1959). They followed Peplau's lead by focusing upon the importance of interpersonal relations. Their work was largely concerned with concept identification, and nurse historians refer to these pioneers as the 'conceptualists' (Meleis, 2007).

One would have thought that six new nursing models in less than a decade would have given ample content for practice, research and education. However, the perpetuation of a desire for new knowledge and innovative ways of looking at old knowledge was unstoppable. This led to a very productive spell in the 1960s. No doubt this was fuelled by the atmosphere of freedom, self-worth and new ideas that permeated 1960s society. So it was that new nurse theorists began to publish their work. Included in this was Faye Abdellah (Abdellah et al, 1960), Ida Orlando (1961), Ernestina Wiedenbach (1964), Martha Levine (1966), Joyce Travelbee (1966) and

Imogene King (1968). Of these formulations Abdellah, Orlando and Travelbee were undoubtedly influenced by Peplau, with the latter two theorists concentrating particularly on psychiatric nursing.

Interestingly, many of these theorists attended Teacher's College at Columbia University in New York and were influenced by the American philosopher, psychologist and educationalist John Dewey (1859–1952). This college became the 'alma mater' for nurse theorists like Peplau, Henderson, Hall, King, Wiedenbach, and Rogers. Abdellah's doctoral dissertation was prepared there under the supervision of Peplau. However, it was not the only seedbed for nursing models. In the mid-1960s, Yale University School of Nursing was given federal funding to identify and examine concepts pertaining to psychiatric nursing. Orlando, who did most of her work there, was the first nurse to discuss the concept of the 'nursing process'.

In the 1960s there appeared to be a production frenzy among US theorists leading to the rapid growth in the number of nursing models produced. However, the 1970s were to see the greatest number of new models. This was probably kick-started when the National League of Nursing specified as an accreditation criterion that nursing curricula should be based upon a conceptual framework. The result was a plethora of models by Callista Roy (1970), Martha Rogers (1970), Betty Neuman (1972), Joan Riehl (1974), Madeline Leininger (1978), Jean Watson (1979), Josephine Paterson (1976) and Margaret Newman (1979). Of these theorists, Neuman, Paterson, Leininger, Watson and Riehl have all specialised and worked extensively in psychiatric nursing, reflecting Peplau's legacy. Other theorists like Roy were influenced by the teaching of people like Dorothy Johnston.

Developing nursing models: Accident or design?

There are two stories that highlight the interesting, yet arguably non-scientific, way in which some of these models were formulated. Callista Roy was kind enough to provide personal communication to the authors on the 'origins' of her fine scholarly work:

I was in a new master's student in paediatric nursing class taught by Dorothy Johnson in 1964. There were no classes in nursing theory and I had not heard about the Johnson model because it was the first day of class. Professor Johnson simply told us that before we got into content on advanced practice in paediatric nursing, we would discuss the goal of nursing. I raised my hand and said that I thought the goal was to promote patient adaptation. I had read one paragraph in a textbook in another class that summer and drew in a light bulb next to the paragraph on adaptation because it stuck me as very related to nursing.

*She asked me, 'What do you mean by that?' So now I have spent
40+ years answering that question. Later I could also identify that my
clinical experience in paediatics and the resilience of children influenced
my insight. Though I never met Harry Helson, I was writing a paper for
my class that semester to expand my ideas, I found a book in the library
that had just come out by Helson on Adaptation Level Theory. I was
looking for a good way to define adaptation and found that work initially
helpful. Fortunately I was a very young graduate student and so have had
many years to work on the theory, including the wonderful opportunity of
implementing it in an undergraduate programme in 1970.*

The second story, also verified in personal communication with Callista
Roy, relates to Betty Neuman and her nursing model. Apparently, Betty Neuman
had initially published her theory in 1972. It was from her work to develop a
grant for a masters' programme on the psychiatric nursing consultation. Her
name was on the list to be invited to the 1978 Nurse Educator Conference
on Nursing Theory in New York City. By accident Margaret Newman was
invited and she said she could take her work on research on activity and time
and address it from a broader theoretical perspective. So Margaret Newman
presented and continues to develop her work to this day. Betty Neuman was
never invited and only found out about it later.

Nursing models: A slow down

In the 1980s in America there was at last a slowing down in the number of
nursing models being developed. Established theorists such as Roy, King,
Watson and Peplau began revising their work and strengthening what they
perceived to be their emerging theories. Meanwhile, new nurse theorists
such as Rosmarie Parse (1981) and Joyce Fitzpatrick (Fitzpatrick and Whall,
1983) formulated their models from the work previously developed by
Martha Rogers (1970). Although Peplau's model had been a template for
those interpersonal theorists that followed, the building of new models on
an older model was an interesting and novel departure in the development
of nursing models.

The evolution of American nursing models between the 1950s and the
1970s was characterised by an adherence to logical positivism where the
hypothetico-deductive view of science was preferred (McKenna, 1997).
Conversely, in the late 1970s and 1980s the phenomenological approach
came into favour reflected in the more humanistic models of Newman
(1979), Parse (1981) and Fitzpatrick (Fitzpatrick and Whall, 1983). This
shift in theoretical approach coincided with the increased appearance of
qualitative methods within nursing research.

British nursing models

As we have seen above, Florence Nightingale began to develop her nursing model in 19th century England. Nonetheless the United Kingdom does not boast a tradition of nursing model development. However, 30 years after Peplau constructed her nursing model, British nurses were being confronted with many of the stimuli that led to the development of American nursing models. These included a disenchantment with the medical model; the arrival of university education for nurses; the establishment academic journals such as the *Journal of Advanced Nursing* and the *International Journal of Nursing Studies*; the quest for professional status; the need to develop a scientific basis for nursing; and the increased expectations and involvement of the patient.

Furthermore, it is important to examine the social context that accompanied the introduction of British nursing models. In the late 1970s and 1980s nursing was undergoing tremendous social change. The move from a traditional task-centred activity to a more patient-focused problem solving approach was a vitally important step for nursing at that time. There was also an increase in the number of graduate and post-graduate nursing degree courses at tertiary education establishments. This had the effect of stimulating an in-depth analysis concerning the appropriateness of the medical and other non-nursing models.

In addition, the patriarchal authority over women and women's work symbolised by the medical model was recognised as having no place in modern nursing. Nurses wished to reject the handmaiden image and be recognised by society as professionals in their own right. In addition, no longer was it legitimate to view patients as passive hosts of a disease process; they became active holistic individuals. Quality assurance programmes were being introduced with an emphasis on consumerism, and individuals were being given more rights. Nurses were also beginning to view care as their central concern rather than looking to the medical model of cure for professional validation. Many believed that patient-centred nursing models were vehicles for actualising new philosophies and models. As a result there followed a flowering of British nursing models. These included the work of Nancy Roper (Roper et al, 1980), Jean McFarlane (1982), Felicity Stockwell (1985), Steve Wright (1986), George Castledine (1986), June Clark (1986), and Jean Minshull (Minshull et al, 1986).

As these British nursing models have grown in number they have been viewed with interest by nurse practitioners and educators alike. Some have been criticised as being in the early stages of development and hence of limited value. It appears that as the number of models increased the attitudes towards them become more varied. In Chapter 1 the perceived benefits of nursing models were outlined. However, there are also perceived limitations.

Limitations of nursing models

Nursing models have not gone without criticism nor have their disadvantages been ignored. Two major limitations have already been alluded to; namely, the belief that nursing models are not specific enough to be regarded as theories and the fact that there are so many nursing models that it is difficult for clinical nurses and nurse practitioners and educators to be familiar with them all.

Many nursing models have been criticised as being jargonistic and cryptic and this has raised their unpopularity with clinicians and their unmanageability at clinical level. There is also the danger that complicated diagrams and neologisms cause widespread confusion not only among practising nurses but also among the public and other health professionals.

Another source of alienation of nursing models has been the emphasis on large amounts of paperwork. As a result the implementation of nursing models in clinical practice is seen by many as a 'paper exercise'. This is not helped by the modern-day emphasis on clinical audit, care planning and clinical governance. It is probable that paperwork would have increased anyway but in many instances nursing models have been blamed for it.

As can be seen above, most existing nursing models have had their origin in the United States. The application of these models to Britain, where there is a different healthcare system, a different nurse educational system and a different values system, poses the question: are these models transferable to nursing practice in Britain? It could be argued that there is nothing wrong with nurses learning about models from other disciplines or other countries but the application of these to patient problems needs careful consideration.

By definition, a nursing model provides a comprehensive overview of the metaparadigm elements. Therefore, assessing a patient using a nursing model can uncover a number of actual and potential problems. In a busy clinical setting the results of such assessment has staffing and skill mix implications. In addition, if a model identifies goals which cannot be met due to lack of time, clinical nurses are likely to become frustrated and demoralised. This may also raise ethical issues: is it morally right to uncover multiple problems in a patient when only a few will be dealt with in the time the patient is in hospital?

We have castigated the medical model for reducing the patient to a set of anatomical parts and physiological systems. However, reductionism can also be a limitation of nursing models. For example, does Roper et al (2000), not reduce patients to 12 activities of living? Does Roy (1970) not reduce patients to four adaptation modes? Does Orem (1995) not reduce patients to a set of self-care needs? Reductionism is reductionism regardless of the theoretical focus or origin.

The goal of most nursing models is to improve nursing care. This inevitably means that such models focus on what nursing ought to be rather than what it currently is. The dilemma faced by practising nurses is if the emphasis is on what ought to be, how can they be useful within the real world of practice? Therefore, those who wish to introduce a conceptual framework into the practical situation may be met by sceptical practitioners who see conceptual frameworks as merely an academic exercise aimed at increasing the complexities of their lives.

Nursing models and nurse education

Most nursing curricula should be underpinned by one or more nursing models. This model should contain the concepts which will identify the discipline's main values and beliefs. It should match the needs of practice. For example, if Orem's self-care model was used to underpin a nursing curriculum, one would expect self-care to permeate all assessments, plans and interventions

Having experience with different models will encourage students to think and reflect more broadly than they would do otherwise. This is an important point but considering the large number of nursing models available, it is unrealistic to expect any one clinical nurse or nurse educator to be familiar with any more than a few of the most popular.

Perhaps there should be an embargo on the formulation of any new nursing models? Rather, efforts should be put into testing and refining those that already exist. While such a moratorium may be popular with clinical nurses it would be difficult to implement. Creative people will continue to formulate models to describe and explain nursing. To stop them from doing so would be wrong. To paraphrase the 19th century politician, Charles Stewart Parnell, (1885), no person, profession or organisation has the right to fix a boundary to the march of a discipline; no one has the right to say this far you should go and no further.

Summary

This chapter shows how Florence Nightingale began to conceptualise nursing in the mid-19th century. She was 'to the manor born' but her work in Scutari began to dignify nursing and led to the development of a highly respected nurse training enterprise. However, in the early 20th century, many of Nightingale's views of nursing were replaced by the medical model. It emphasised cure rather than care and simplistically envisaged individuals as broken machines that required repair. The medical model held sway for over 50 years and in some cases vestiges of it remain. However, it was a disenchantment with the medical model that led Hildegard Peplau to formulate her model of nursing in the early 1950s. This encouraged other fledgling theorists and in a matter of a generation there were a number of nursing models on both sides of the Atlantic. Accepting that these models aim to make the patient's experience of illness more bearable, they are not without their perceived limitations.

References

Abdellah FG, Beland IL, Martin A, Matheney RV (1960) *Patient Centred Approaches to Nursing*. Macmillan, New York

Castledine G (1986) A stress adaptation model. In: Kershaw B, Salvage J (eds) *Models for Nursing*. John Wiley & Sons, Chichester

Clark J (1986) A model for health visiting. In: Kershaw B, Salvage J (eds) *Models for Nursing*. John Wiley & Sons, Chichester

Dickens C (1866) *The Life and Adventures of Martin Chuzzlewit*. Chapman and Hall, London

Fitzpatrick JJ, Whall AL (1983) *Conceptual Models of Nursing: Analysis and Application*. Brady Co, Maryland

Hall L (1959) *Nursing - What is it?* Virginia State Nurses Association, Virginia

Henderson V, Harmer B (1955) *Textbook of the Principles and Practices of Nursing*. 5th edn. Macmillan, New York

Johnson DE (1959) The nature of a science of nursing. *Nursing Outlook* 7: 291–4

King I (1968) A conceptual frame of reference for nursing. *Nursing Research* 17(1): 27–31

Leininger MM (1978) *Transcultural Nursing: Concepts, Theories, and Practices*. John Wiley & Sons, New York

Levine ME (1994) Some further thoughts on the ethics of nursing rhetoric. In: Kikuchi F, Simmons H (eds) *Developing a Philosophy of Nursing*. Sage, Thousand Oaks

McFarlane JK (1982) *Nursing: A Paradigm of Caring*. Unpublished Paper. Ethical Issues in Caring. University of Manchester

McKenna HP (1997) *Nursing Models and Theories*. Routledge, London

McKenna HP, Thompson D, Watson R (2007) Health care assistants: An oxymoron? *International Journal of Nursing Studies* 44(8): 1283–4

Meleis AI (2007) *Theoretical Nursing: Development and Progress*. 4th edn. Lippincott Williams and Wilkins, Philadelphia

Minshull J, Ross K, Turner J (1986) The human needs model of nursing. *Journal of Advanced Nursing* 11: 643–9

Neuman B (1995) *The Neuman Systems Model*. 3rd edn. Appleton and Lange, Norwalk

Newman MA (1979) *Theory Development in Nursing*. 3rd edn. FA Davis & Co, Philadelphia

Nightingale F (1859/1980) *Notes on Nursing: What It Is and What It Is Not*. Churchill Livingstone, Edinburgh

Norris CM (1970) *Proceedings from the 2nd Annual Nursing Theory Conference*. University of Kansas, Kansas

Orem DE (1959) *Guides for Development of Curriculae for the Education of Practical Nurses*. US Dept of Health, Education and Welfare, Washington DC

Orem DE (1995) *Nursing: Concepts of Practice*. 5th edn. McGraw Hill, New York

Orlando I (1961) *The Dynamic Nurse Patient Relationship. Function, Process, and Principles*. GP Putnam & Sons, New York

Parnell CS (1885) Speech at Cork, Ireland. Engraved on the Parnell Monument, Parnell Square, Dublin

Parse RR (1981) *Man-Living-Health: A Theory of Nursing*. John Wiley & Sons, New York

Parsons T (1952) *The Social System*. London, Tavistock Publications.

Peplau HE (1952) *Interpersonal Relations in Nursing*. New York: G.P.Putnam & Sons

Peplau HE (1987) Nursing science: A historical perspective. In: Parse RR (ed) *Nursing Science: Major Paradigms, Theories and Critiques*. WB Saunders Co, Philadelphia

Riehl JP (1974) The Riehl interactional model. In: Riehl JP, Roy C (eds) *Conceptual Models in Nursing Practice*. Appleton-Century-Crofts, New York

Rogers ME (1970) *An Introduction to a Theoretical Basis of Nursing*. FA Davis & Co, Philadelphia

Roper N, Logan N, Tierney A (1980) *Elements of Nursing*. Churchill Livingstone, Edinburgh

Roper N, Logan W, Tierney AJ (2000) *The Roper-Logan-Tierney Model of Nursing Based on Activities of Living*. Churchill-Livingstone, Edinburgh

Roy C (1970) Adaptation - A Conceptual Framework for Nursing. *Nursing Outlook* **18**(3): 42–5

Stockwell F (1985) *The Nursing Process in Psychiatric Nursing*. Croom Helm, London

Travelbee J (1966) *Interpersonal Aspects of Nursing*. FA Davis, Philadelphia

Walshe JJ (1929) *The History of Nursing*. Kennedy & Sons, New York

Wiedenbach E (1964) *Clinical Nursing: A Helping Art*. Springer Publication Company, New York

Wright SG (1986) *Building and Using a Model of Nursing*. Edward Arnold, London:

CHAPTER 4

Hildegard Peplau's Interpersonal Relations Model

Sometimes described as the 'mother of psychiatric nursing', Peplau has had a profound effect on nursing; an effect that clearly transcends her specialism of psychiatric nursing (Haber, 2000). As one of the earliest authors of and subsequently pioneers in nursing theory and models, her 'Interpersonal Relations Model' (sometimes referred to as a developmental model – see Pearson and Vaughan, 1986) not only served as a conceptual template for subsequent nursing theorists (and their associated models), it was also (and remains) a major, seminal contribution to nursing science. Indeed, if contemporary references to the nurse–patient relationship are anything to go by, then her legacy is alive and well, if not thriving, in the 21st century. Furthermore, her model has been used as the theoretical underpinning for a variety of psychiatric nursing textbooks over the years (see, for example, Rawlins et al, 1993; Varcarolis et al, 2006) and as the basis for psychiatric nursing curricula (see Stenberg College, 2008).

Her original 1952 book, *Interpersonal Relations in Nursing*, revised and republished in 1988, illustrates the world view and beliefs that underpin her model, the rudiments of the model, phases of the nurse–patient relationship, and the different roles of nursing. In terms of the correct term to use when describing Peplau's work, examination of the literature shows inconsistent usage. Peplau herself probably used the term 'theory' more than she used the word 'model' although in her own words, she denied that 'theory' was the best term; preferring instead the less succinct phrase 'a set of concepts, a framework that can be applied to various kinds of nursing situations'. Others have used the term 'conceptual model' (Riehl and Roy, 1980; Pearson and Vaughan, 1986; Aggleton and Chalmers, 2000) and books that have been written about nursing models (e.g. Pearson and Vaughan, 1986; Aggleton and Chalmers, 2000) each contain a chapter focused on Peplau's nursing 'model'. While 'model' may or may not be the most appropriate term to describe Peplau's work, in the interests of symmetry and consistency of this book, we have chosen to use it.

Bearing in mind that Peplau's seminal book was originally published in

1952, it is perhaps not surprising that she drew significantly on the work of prominent scholars of her time (and earlier). One does not have to look very far into Peplau's work to see the influence of 'humanists' (among others and to a greater and lesser extent), Frieda Fromm-Reichman (1889–1957), Harry Sullivan (1953) and Abraham Maslow (1954). As a result, her work underscores the individual worth of human beings, the need to treat all people with dignity and respect and the capacity that each person has for personal development and growth. She further posits that the central feature of nursing practice is the nurse–patient relationship (Peplau, 1991). Also, study of Peplau's work will lead the reader to the inescapable conclusion that her work was highly influenced by Freud (1936) and his psychodynamic ideas. Indeed, while Freud and his ideas may have fallen out of favour, such was the influence of this work on Peplau that she makes frequent references to her model of 'psychodynamic nursing'. Further evidence of the influence of Freud can be detected in Peplau's emphasis on anxiety and how there is a universal human need to harness the energy that comes from tension and anxiety. It can also be seen in Peplau's reference to the importance of patterns, pattern recognition and pattern integration.

Interestingly, although the original version was produced prior to Kuhn's (1962) classic work on metaparadigms, if one reads her text carefully, Peplau can be seen to speak to each of the four Khunian metaparadigms of person, health, nursing and environment; albeit implicitly in some cases and she says more about some metaparadigms than she does about others.

Nursing

What is nursing? For Peplau, this is a question that every student should ask for themselves in order that they can become aware of what is involved in this phenomenon we call nursing. Furthermore, Peplau argues that these important musings lead to enlightenment about what nursing is currently, but equally importantly, what nursing ought to be. Peplau (1988: 5) asserts that nursing is, firstly, a process; she continues:

> *By this we mean that its serial and goal-directed nature demands certain steps, actions, operations or performances that occur between the individual who does the nursing and the person who is nursed.*

Moreover, from this one can assert that it is an *interpersonal process* (original emphasis) and most often (although we would add, not always) a *therapeutic one*. For Peplau, nursing then is inescapably a human relationship between the person(s) in need of health services and the nurse; a specifically educated person who is thus able to acknowledge and act in response to these identified needs. Nursing accordingly requires an initial effort directed towards attempting to understand the nature of the need (problem). For Peplau, while nursing has changed over the years and will continue to do so, it is concerned with health (or wellness) – not illness or sickness. Her prophetic comments that, 'curative methods in nursing have tended to supersede developmental or preventative ones' (1988: 6), are just as relevant and applicable to 21st century nursing as they were when the book was first written over 60 years ago. (Indeed, an argument can easily be made that this is more the case today in most developed – or Western – healthcare systems see, for example, President Barack Obama's Health Care Plan, recovered 2009, where it is acknowledged that there has been significant under-investment in preventative healthcare and public health [primary prevention] measures.) Peplau continues by purporting that nursing requires a series of operations that are geared to bring about the achievement of health. She also declares that nursing is a function; a maturing force and an educative instrument. Interestingly, Peplau maintains that nursing involves helping or aiding individuals (or family/community) to use their own capacities to bring about positive changes in their lives. There is a clear sense here then of Peplau arguing that nursing involves promoting and facilitating the development of the person in need of help; that nursing is often 'doing with' rather than 'doing for'; that nursing involves helping people learn new ways of responding to their health problems. Furthermore, Peplau (1988) is clear in believing that nursing is not a static concept; it develops in light of the times, sociopolitical change, adaptations in culture, etc.

Peplau (1988) describes a particularly psychodynamic view of nursing, indeed she often refers to psychodynamic nursing. As a result, her model makes reference to unresolved conflicts from early life, to how human behaviour and relationships are shaped by both conscious and unconscious influences, to recognising the influence of the past on oneself in the present (the 'here and now'), and to how nurses can help patients replace these previous experiences with views that promote growth, learning and development in the person. Peplau (1988: 16) summarises her conceptualisation of nursing:

Nursing is a significant, therapeutic, interpersonal process. It functions co-operatively with other human processes that make health possible for individuals in communities. In specific situations in which a professional health team offers health services, nurses participate in the organisation of conditions that facilitate ongoing tendencies in human organisms. Nursing is an educative instrument, a maturing force, that aims to promote forward movement of personality in the direction of creative, constructive, productive, personal and community living.

Health

For Peplau (1988: 12) the concept of health had not been clearly defined, although she offers a tentative definition:

> *....a word symbol that implies forward movement of personality and other ongoing human processes in the direction of creative, constructive, productive, personal and community living.*

Peplau appears to say more about health problems than she does about health. She furthermore appears less focused on or orientated to, for want of a better expression, heavily biomedically influenced constructs (and subsequent definitions) of health; and for the authors, this is refreshingly dissimilar to many nursing models. Health is related to satisfying or meeting the person's needs, goals and security (Peplau, 1988: 78) and is the primary goal of nursing. For Peplau (1988: 80), who is clearly drawing on Maslow (1954) here, the healthy person is one who has his/her basic needs met. However, Peplau again draws heavily on psychodynamic ideas to suggest that a person's sense of being unhealthy in the 'here and now' can often result from unmet needs from the past. Peplau (1988: 82) also speaks of a person living in,

> *a state of unstable equilibrium (i.e. physiological, psychological and social fluidity) and life is the process of striving in the direction of stable equilibrium, i.e. a fixed pattern that is never reached until death.*

It should be noted, however, that the term 'equilibrium' has been criticised by some authors (e.g. Forchuck, 1991a, b) suggesting that the term is more congruent with closed systems rather than open systems (i.e. a system that interacts with the environment).

Peplau (1988: 18) wrote of 'felt needs' as indicators of the need for nursing; felt needs as health problems. From this one can deduce that for Peplau health is equated with no felt needs; no health problems. She purports (1988: 14) that health is promoted or supported by psychobiological processes, that of self-repair and self-development.

> *General conditions that are likely to lead to health – the interpersonal environment, biological needs for fluids, vitamins, endocrine substances and the like. Repair or removal of any impediment to physiological functioning, dietary manipulations and supportive medications.*

Peplau clearly links health with personal holistic growth and development.

Given that to be human is to live in this constantly unstable environment wherein people face new challenges, new stressors, new 'felt needs', new experiences, a healthy person then is one who responds to these challenges and stimuli and consequently grows and develops.

Persons

For Peplau, people are human beings who inhabit unstable environments. In so doing, they exist in a state of physiological, psychological and sociological flux; people then are dynamic and capable of (if not actually required to) engage in change and growth. Thus, for Peplau, persons or humans have an innate capacity for development and growth. In offering such views, Peplau clearly draws on several humanistic writers (of her time) such as Fromm-Reichman, Sullivan and Maslow, and further evidence of these influences on Peplau are evident whereby she acknowledges and regards the uniqueness of each human as sacrosanct. This uniqueness is comprised of individual experiences, beliefs, expectations and patterns of interpersonal relations. But, perhaps paradoxically, while the uniqueness of the individual is recognised, Peplau (1988) also argues that every person has 'felt needs', and that they are either instinctual or have been acquired in the process of socialisation (1988: 73), so people are not, *ipso facto*, healthy. Illness for Peplau is viewed as an opportunity for growth; a learning experience, and yet people seldom have the personalised knowledge and/or awareness of the felt need to fully understand it. Accordingly, people seek assistance on the basis of a felt need, a need that is felt but poorly understood.

In some of her later writings, (see Peplau, 1997) Peplau develops some of her earlier ideas about persons or humans and purports that part of being human is to require interpersonal relationships; that given the challenges of the 21st century, it is all the more necessary for people to engage with other people in meaningful ways. Also, in Peplau's view, to be a person is to encounter difficulties in interpersonal relationships throughout one's life, albeit to varying degrees and intensities.

Environment

Examination of Peplau's various works appears to indicate that she says less about the environment than she does about the other metaparadigms of nursing. Although, if one regards the 'interpersonal environment' as one component of the larger metaparadigm of 'environment', then this may not be the case, because for Peplau (1988, 1991) the interpersonal environment between the patient and the nurse is critical; it is for Peplau the heart of nursing. In Peplau's view then, processes such as communication and pattern integration might be thought of as part of this paradigm since they are key concepts within the interpersonal environment. For example, Peplau (1987) describes how earlier, learned patterns within the patient regarding personal withdrawal can be challenged (and thus space for new patterns is created) by an interested and exploratory nurse.

Although perhaps few in evidence, remarks concerning the physical and sociopolitical environment can be found, for example, Peplau (1988) purports that nursing can do more than it is doing now and thus widen the types of environments where nursing occurs. Indeed, and while the historical period of time when Peplau made these remarks should be considered here, the authors would argue that, despite the progress made since this time, these comments are just as relevant today as they were when they were first uttered. There is a great deal more that nurses could be doing, particularly if they aspire to transformational leadership, and thus take an active and participatory role in policy formation and critique (see for example, Sofarelli and Brown, 1998; Sullivan and Decker, 2001; Cutcliffe and Wieck, 2008). Peplau (1997) indeed refers to such a development in nursing and its associated change in 'environment' when she discusses the social changes that have occurred over recent years and the introduction of primary nursing. Perhaps this reflects further Peplau's views on how people inhabit unstable environments. Society then, for Peplau, is similarly capable of development and growth just as humans are.

An additional element of the sociopolitical environment that Peplau (1988: 12) refers to is that of the multi-disciplinary team environment. Nurses, she writes, are by no means alone in sharing the responsibility with other professional (healthcare) workers, for 'stating criteria for desirable living and for working out policies and plans for achieving conditions to make health possible'.

Further into her key text, Peplau qualifies her remarks when she states,

The hospital ward is a social context in which the patient can be aided to grow in the direction of health requires investigation of the into conditions it provides that facilitate promotion of physical, emotional and social well-being. Nurses have primary responsibility for development and improvement of this social context so that growth can occur. *(Emphasis added)*

It is therefore interesting to note that Peplau regards it as the primary responsibility of nursing and not any other disciplinary or professional healthcare group to develop the environment, as the social context is part of this environment, as a mechanism for effective nursing. It is the view of the authors that this sociopolitical orientated aspect of Peplau's theory is seldom identified in other texts and thus such literature misses a key aspect of Peplau's broader views of what nursing is and what nurses should be doing.

Nursing roles

Peplau (1988, 1997) asserts that nurses need to occupy and act in a variety of different roles – some of which nurses choose to adopt, some of which clients usher nurses into, and some which society and/or the professional literature suggest nurses should be adopting.

Stranger

On all first encounters with a new client, the nurse's initial role, Peplau declares, is that of stranger. As a result, as a stranger the nurse should demonstrate and communicate the same qualities and courtesies that one should offer as a matter of course to any new guest. For Peplau, these qualities/courtesies are:

- Respect.
- Positive interest.
- Acceptance of the individual just the way he/she is.
- Treating the person as an emotionally able person (until there is evidence to treat him/her otherwise).

Unless the nurse, Peplau suggests, is able to communicate respect and a sense of mutual interest, the relationship is unlikely to develop any sense of trust and will be 'stuck' in the stage of orientation.

Resource person

Nurses can and need to be an abundant source of knowledge and information for the person they work with, and thus will need to supply specific answers to questions. The specific educational background and preparation that nurses have, Peplau purports, equips them to be able to answer these often 'technical' questions; for example, how to change a dressing or what is the range of 'normal/healthy' blood pressure readings. Interestingly, Peplau (1988: 48) also notes that all questions need to be answered immediately and some musings or questions need to be grappled with and explored by individuals themselves. Peplau argues that this discerning and thoughtful approach is a feature of competent nursing (and here the authors would argue that this is a feature of increasing competence and excellence in practice – *à la* Benner's (1984) work on the development of nurses from novice to expert; a tendency to try and answer all the client's questions immediately is likely to be indicative of less expert practice), that these expert practitioners will learn to discriminate between questions that need answers immediately and other questions that have developmental value if they are left for the client to think about and work through.

Teacher

For Peplau, the teaching role in nursing combines elements of each of the other nursing roles. It always begins from what the person knows already and from there focuses on the person's interest in gaining *medical* (our emphasis) information. (While the authors would argue health-related rather than medical knowledge would be a more appropriate term, perhaps the particular time the first book was written might account for this.) Interestingly, Peplau qualifies her position of this teaching role when she points out that it does not refer to a didactic or traditional teaching role, but is more concerned with experiential learning (*à la* Dewey, 2007). Accordingly, in Peplau's model, the nurse's teaching role is inherently concerned with development; or, to paraphrase, the acquisition or development of new knowledge, skills and/or abilities that enable what Peplau (1988: 48) refers to as 'open-ended outcomes'.

Surrogate

With another clear reference to psychodynamic thinking, Peplau purports that nurses will be cast in the role of surrogate by clients, often without the clients' awareness. In place of relating and responding to individual nurses, clients subsequently find themselves relating and responding to nurses as if they were the other person. As a result, Peplau notes that patients' feelings experienced in earlier relationships will subsequently influence what they expect from their relationships with the nurse. By way of an example, if the person places the nurse in the role of surrogate father, and the previous experience of the father is one personified by unwanted attempts at control resulting in frustration and hostility in the person, the likelihood is that the person will react with frustration and hostility towards the nurse. Yet in all these situations, Peplau argues that it is important for the nurse to accept the person as he or she is, to accept whatever feelings the person expresses towards the nurse and such acceptance can then help lead the person to understand the differences between the earlier experience and the nurse. It is in allowing the person to re-experience these older feelings in new situations, but this time in the interpersonal climate of acceptance and attention, that promotes personality development. For Peplau, the ability of the nurse to

Least intensive   **Most intensive**

←——→

Using counselling   Working in a   Structured,
skills   counselling way   sessional counselling
                                                       with trained/educated
                                                       psychotherapists

Figure 1.1 Continuum of counselling activity.

be able to recognise what surrogate roles the person is casting the nurse in, identifying the particular interpersonal difficulties that the person is working through in casting the nurse in this role, and sustaining a working relationship that develops awareness in the person during these times, are key nursing skills.

Counsellor

Given Peplau's views of nursing as a developmental process it is not surprising that she views the counselling role of the nurse as one concerned with helping patients discover the nature of their problems (or felt needs), revealing the difficulties they have to face (and overcome) rather than suppressing or ignoring them. Peplau describes this counselling as the nurse working with patients in order to satisfy unmet needs from their past through continuing growth and development (in the 'here and now'). For Peplau, all these counselling functions are driven and thus determined by the particular nurse–client relationship; or, to paraphrase, they are driven by the particular experiences that clients need to undergo that will lead to their health and development.

It is important to note that Peplau makes a very clear distinction between what she describes as the nurse's counselling role and the counselling role (and practice) more commonly associated with psychotherapists. For the authors, this can be further explained by thinking of the continuum of psychotherapeutic work (see *Figure 1.1*), with Peplau's counselling role being analogous to 'working in a counselling way'. In this role, Peplau purports that the nurse needs to help individuals become aware of the conditions that are required for health, then provide these conditions (whenever possible), then help individuals recognise the threats to their health and use the nursing encounter (for Peplau, an interpersonal event) to facilitate their learning and development. Peplau's counselling role is concerned with the way nurses respond to demands made upon them and is a process concerned with helping individuals gain insight and understanding into their problems and, importantly, how and why they are responding to these problems in a certain way. Thus, the process is about exploring how individuals feel about themselves and what they are experiencing; how they feel about what is happening to them.

Leader

In Peplau's view, leadership is a function in all situations and she argues further that nurses must demonstrate leadership as a function of democratic living. This leadership is enacted in more places than the individual clinical scenario; it is also operationalised at national and international levels. While Peplau does outline three different types of leadership – democratic, autocratic and *laissez-faire* – her emphasis is clearly on democratic leadership. In such an approach to leadership, the agenda (and power) are shared between participants; policies and goals are co-determined, and courses of action are discussed openly. However, Peplau does add a cautionary caveat noting that current practice in nursing still has some way to go before it achieves truly democratic nursing. Nevertheless, such a leadership role is clearly bound up once more with encouraging the development of the person; of working alongside the person rather than doing unto.

Peplau's phases of the nurse–patient relationship

In her original work Peplau (1988) described four phases of the nurse–patient relationship and several authors have previously likened these phases to the four stages of the nursing process (see Pearson and Vaughan, 1986; Aggleton and Chalmers, 2000) (although it is fair to note that these authors also highlight differences between Peplau's phases and the stages of the nursing process). Although in her later work and in other important contributions to the development of this model these have been presented as having two (Forchuk and Brown, 1989; Forchuk, 1991a, b) or three phases (Peplau, 1997). Peplau's original design will be used here to describe each of the four phases. Peplau herself asserts that these four phases are seldom experienced as a linear sequence and as entirely separate, discrete phases. Not only do these phases overlap and interlock with one another but the process of progression through these phases is more chaotic; with both 'forwards' and 'backwards' movements between the phases occurring. The authors argue that the metaphor that perhaps best captures the nature of this multi-direction progression is that of the movement of the tide (see also Cutcliffe, 2004). So while there is a progressive and gradual movement of the tide in one direction, this is not a uni-directional, linear movement; individual waves move backwards and forwards.

Orientation phase

Peplau (1997) declares that of all her phases, the orientation phase is more driven by or initialised by nurses. It is nurses who should first take the initiative and identify themselves, it is nurses who set the parameters in terms of time available; and while nurses must seek important yet personal information from the person (i.e. initial assessment interview, history taking) the person does not need any personal information about the nurse. Nurses' attention needs to be focused on the patient, listening and hearing what is said. Peplau purports that at this time, the nurse needs to ask 'who, what, where, when' type questions to encourage patients to tell their story. In addition to garnering this key assessment information (and thus the similarity with the 'assessment' stage of the nursing process) Peplau (1997: 164) states that:

The aims are to set the tone for further interactions and to convey professional respect and receptivity for the patient ... it is the time to begin to know the patient as a person.

In so doing, the orientation phase is associated with the beginnings of the development of trust between the nurse and the patient. In this phase individuals become aware of a 'felt need', they realise that they have a need for healthcare and that as a result, professional healthcare services should be sought. While individuals may be aware that they have a need, they simultaneously lack awareness and/or knowledge of the need to fully understand it. For Peplau, seeking assistance under these circumstances is a key element of the orientation phase and also importantly is the first step in a dynamic learning experience from which personal growth can occur. Peplau stresses that during this phase, individuls will often provide the lead on how they visualise or conceptualise the problem and that this will allow the nurse to establish where gaps in their understanding exist. However, it is only by means of hearing the person's story; by listening a lot and saying little that this learning opportunity for the person can occur. Peplau contends that nursse can adopt any (all) of their nursing roles and so aid this process of clarification. This then enables individuals to recognise and understand the nature of their felt need and importantly, also recognise their need for help to address that need. As a result, both the person and the nurse come to learn the nature of the felt need. Although Peplau acknowledges that this orientating to the problem can be a complex task, she adds that it is essential to enlist individuals in identifying and assessing their problems; that given that addressing these problems is of great concern to them it is necessary to engage them as active participants. This is achieved by the nurse responding unconditionally; that is, Peplau (1988: 29) states:

Making no demands upon the patient to satisfy her own needs rather than his own, orientating the patient towards focusing on the problem, will permit the patient to express his feelings so that he can become aware of what they are.

Peplau also describes how the orientation phase is concerned with nurses assisting individuals to harness the energy that arises as a result of the anxiety and tension experienced by them in response to their felt need. Peplau underscores the importance of this particular nursing intervention in the orientation phase when she argues that if this anxiety/tension is ignored (during the frenetic activity of being admitted), then this will set the tone for the remainder of the nurse–patient relationship.

Identification phase

Peplau (1988) suggests that when individuals have clarified and gained some deeper understanding of their felt need, combined with a sense of what they feel this situation can offer them, they will then respond selectively to the people who appear to be able to offer them the help they need. At this point, the nurse–patient relationship is moving into the identification phase. Interestingly, this identification phase is less concerned with further identification of the problem (as the name might suggest) but is more of a reference to the psychodynamic process of identification; a process of identifying with and subsequently relating to the nurse. It is this process and/or feeling of being able to relate to others, in a way that enables the expression of underlying wishes, Peplau (1988) argues, that is possible in and necessary for nursing situations. Furthermore, it is during what Peplau (1988: 31) refers to as 'the natural vehicles of nursing care, e.g. bathing, feeding, giving enemas', etc., that this identification and sense of relatedness can be fostered. Crucially, these activities, which, for some are often regarded as basic functions or indeed a task that needs to be accomplished before moving onto the next task (Thompson et al, 2000), then take on a whole new meaning. The task itself then, for Peplau, becomes secondary to the nexus that is established during these activities.

Persons in this phase will have an individual response to this venture, often including the expression of emotion, especially if trust is being established and the person feels secure and safe in the care of the nurse. Peplau is adamant that when the nurse permits/enables individuals to express whatever they are feeling and still get all the nursing care they need, then individuals are free to experience the 'illness/care episode' as a time for personal growth, development and something that will strengthen the positive forces in their personality. The nurse then needs to further develop the nurse–patient relationship so that it encourages forward movement (or development) of the person's personality and psychological make-up. In so doing, Peplau (1988) predicates that earlier (childhood) experiences and feelings of powerlessness and helplessness within the person can be superseded (replaced) by experiences and feelings of creativeness, spontaneity and productivity.

Exploitation (working) phase

Peplau's (1988) exploitation phase, later described as a sub-phase of the 'working' phase (Forchuck, 1991a, b; Peplau, 1997) occurs when individuals are able identify with a nurse who is able to understand their particular interpersonal relations. When this occurs, patients are open to making full use of the services offered to them. For Peplau (1997), the working phase, being an amalgamation of her original identification and exploitation phases, is where the work gets done. (This amalgamation of two of her original phases into the working phase occurred because Peplau and others recognised that relationships move back and forwards – as we alluded to earlier – as new problems are discovered and subsequently worked through.) For Peplau this willingness to make use of all the services available is contingent upon patients feeling safe, comfortable and well cared for and feeling like participating members (rather than passive recipients). Furthermore, while patients can (and should) make use of all the services available to them, Peplau (1988) writes that they will also be identifying and orientating themselves to new goals, including those related to lessening their dependence on the nurse and the healthcare system, i.e. going back home, returning to work, re-establishing relationships.

Once more Peplau draws heavily on psychodynamic theory and writing in order to describe and explain some of the key interpersonal processes that are occurring in this stage. This apparent paradox between utilising all the services available and yet at the same time striving for and increasing their independence from the nurse is for Peplau analogous to the dependence/independence struggle associated with teenagers. Peplau (1988: 38) describes it thus:

The main difficulty seems to be that of striving to strike a balance between a need to be dependent, as during serious illness, and a need to be independent, such as following recovery. Many patients experience these opposite feelings as conflict, vacillating between them and being unable to decide the direction in which they wish to move.

Peplau (1997) is adamant that during this phase the focus needs to be on patients' reactions to illness and on their work towards developing their understanding of themselves, their current health condition and what new challenges (in terms of personal growth and development) this condition makes of them. Nurses need to adopt any number of Peplau's (1988) previously discussed nursing roles, as they help keep the patients' focus on the work that needs to be done in their own interests; although it is perhaps the case that Peplau (1997) draws particular attention to the roles of teacher, counsellor and resource person. The principle, Peplau (1997) asserts, is for the nurse to struggle with the problem – not the patient. Interventions when the nurse is operating in the counsellor role, Peplau (1997) insists, serve the purpose of facilitating greater self-awareness and self-understanding in the patient. This is achieved by means of the nurse's use of investigative inquiry and active listening as the patient continues to 'tell his or her story'.

Resolution phase

Peplau's (1988) resolution stage, sometimes referred to as the 'termination phase', is concerned with summarising the progress that the patient has made and with achieving a sense of closure (Peplau, 1997). Peplau (1988) declared that this resolution stage should occur when the health problem is resolved; she however qualifies these remarks by stating that this resolution is actually more of a psychological phenomenon than being concerned with medical (physical) recovery. Peplau's final phase of the nurse–patient relationship is also concerned with a gradual freeing of the identification with the helper (i.e. nurses). She describes this as a freeing process where the patient begins to stand alone and she purports that this can only be achieved when all of the other phases have been worked through. Peplau (1988: 40) emphasises that this is most likely to be achieved if, throughout the therapeutic relationship, conditions are provided where patients can organise their actions so that they want to be free for more productive social relationships. For Peplau, this phase includes the requirement for nurses to reflect on the relationship they have engaged in and for patients to reflect on their 'illness' experience and weave these meanings into their lives. It also includes the need for the dyad to consider and plan for alternative forms of support.

Further evidence of the non-linear and overlapping nature of these phases is exemplified by Peplau's writing about the preparation for the termination of the relationship, which does not start in this phase, but should start in the previous 'exploitation' phase. Nevertheless, these terminations or endings can be protracted and continue until all plans have been fully implemented and ends when there are no more nurse–patient encounters arranged.

Clinical application of Peplau's model

Even a cursory examination of the extant literature will indicate that attempts have been made to apply Peplau's model in a variety of nursing situations and specialty areas (see below). In addition, such a review would indicate, we would argue, that Cheryl Forchuk has perhaps been foremost in operationalising Peplau's model into practice. In no way are we demeaning the scholarly contributions from other authors (such as the work of Reynolds), but Forchuk has a 20-year history of this endeavour. Accordingly, for our principle example of the clinical application of Peplau's model we draw on this work, most especially Forchuk and Brown's (1989) instrument (i.e. transitional discharge model) for measuring and determining the phases of the nurse–patient relationship. Our clinical example of the application subsequently includes tables for each phase of Peplau's model. Please see *Tables 4.1* to *4.5*. We follow this with a review of other literature that has attempted to apply and/or operationalise Peplau's model in a variety of clinical/empirical ways.

Forchuk and Brown (1989) suggest that their instrument acts as a pictorial guide that can help in monitoring the development of the nurse–patient relationship as it provides a brief summary of the principal actions, behaviours and/or roles, of both the patient and the nurse, that are particularly associated with each of the phases of the relationship. As a result, by determining to what degree these actions, behaviours and roles are occurring, nurses are better able to judge what phase of the relationship they are in. Forchuk and Brown (1989) report that the instrument appears to provide an accurate assessment of the nurse–patient relationship based on the observable behaviours of the patient and the nurse.

For our clinical case example, we have drawn on a real client, although all details and data have been changed in order to maintain the client's complete confidentiality.

Applications and measures of Peplau's model in clinical practice

Morrison et al (1996) report on a research study that attempted to operationalise Peplau's model in the work roles of psychiatric nursing, in part as a means of further verifying the notion of different nursing roles. Data were collected by audiotaping 62 interactions between nurses and adults, children or adolescent psychiatric patients. This was followed by a content analysis to identify roles that were in addition to those previously described by Peplau. Not only is this a fine example of the application of Peplau's model, but it also attempts to verify, expand and develop her model.

Table 4.1: Clinical example of application of Peplau's model. Forchuck's transitional discharge model

Phases of the therapeutic relationship

Mutual withdrawal	Grappling	Orientation	Working phase	Resolution phase
Client				
• Forgets appointment/ planned times • Cannot recall who nurse/service provider is • Unaware if nurse/service provider is available • Content kept superficial • Actively avoids nurse/ service provider	• Frequent changes of topics and approach • Increasing frustration • Sense of lack of connection • Begins to dread meetings	• Seeks assistance • Conveys educative needs • Asks questions • Tests parameters • Shares pre-conceptions and expectations due to past experience	• Identifies problems • Aware of time • Responds to help • Identifies with PP • Recognises and explores feelings • Fluctuates dependence, independence and interdependence in therapeutic relationship • Increases focal attention • Changes appearance (for better or worse) • Understands purpose of meeting • Maintains continuity between sessions (process and content) • Testing manoeuvres decrease • Increase focal attention • Makes full use of services • Identifies new goals • Rapid shifts in behaviour; dependent–independent • Exploitative behaviour • Realistic exploitation • Self-directing • Develops skills in interpersonal relationships and problem solving	• Abandons old needs • Aspires to new goals • Becomes independent of helping person • Applies new problem-solving skills • Maintains changes in style of communication and interaction • Positive changes in view of self • Integrates illness • Exhibits ability to stand alone

Service provider

• No time for client meetings • Client meetings very short if they occur at all • Focus on instrumental tasks • Decision that client is atypical of usual relationship • Avoids client contact	• Frequent changes of therapeutic approach • Sense of lack of connection • Increasing frustration • Length of meetings vary • Place of meetings vary	• Respond to emergency • Practice non-directive listening • Focus client's energies • Clarify preconceptions and expectations	• Maintain separate identity • Unconditional acceptance • Help express needs, feelings • Assess and adjust to needs • Provide information • Provide experiences that diminish feelings of helplessness • Do not allow anxiety to overwhelm client • Help focus on cues • Help client develop responses to cues • Use word stimuli	• Continue assessment • Meet needs as they emerge • Understand reason for shifts in behaviour • Initiate rehabilitative plans • Reduce anxiety • Identify positive factors • Help plan for total needs • Facilitate forward movement of personality • Deal with therapeutic impasse	• Sustain relationship as long as patient feels necessary • Promote family interaction • Assist with goal setting • Teach preventive measures • Utilise community agencies • Teach self-care • Terminate relationship

Note: Phases are overlapping

MW	GR	O	WP	RP

Mark on the scale where check marks are concentrated within the table

Checklists designed to assist in evaluating phase

Table 4.2: Clinical example of Peplau's model at the relationship stage of mutual withdrawal

Phases of the therapeutic relationship

Mutual withdrawal	Grappling	Orientation	Working phase	Resolution phase
Client				
• Forgets appointment/ planned times: *The patient failed to show up for his scheduled appointment* • Cannot recall who nurse/service provider is: *During our subsequent telephone call, the patient had to be reminded who is was and what my role was* • Unaware if nurse/ service provider available: *The patient remembered that he was supposed to meet with someone from the mental health services but couldn't recall who* • Content kept	• Frequent changes of topics and approach • Increasing frustration • Sense of lack of connection • Begins to dread meetings	• Seeks assistance • Conveys educative needs • Asks questions • Tests parameters • Shares pre-conceptions and expectations due to past experience	• Identifies problems • Aware of time • Responds to help • Identifies with PP • Recognises and explores feelings • Fluctuates dependence, independence and interdependence in therapeutic relationship • Increases focal attention • Changes appearance (for better or worse) • Understands purpose of meeting • Maintains continuity between sessions (process and content) • Testing manoeuvres decrease • Increase focal attention • Makes full use of services • Identifies new goals • Rapid shifts in behaviour; dependent–independent • Exploitative behaviour • Realistic exploitation • Self-directing • Develops skills in interpersonal relationships and problem solving • Displays changes in manner of communication	• Abandons old needs • Aspires to new goals • Becomes independent of helping person • Applies new problem-solving skills • Maintains changes in style of communication and interaction • Positive changes in view of self • Integrates illness • Exhibits ability to stand alone

			(more open, flexible)	• Sustain relationship as long as patient feels necessary • Promote family interaction • Assist with goal setting • Teach preventive measures • Utilise
		• Maintain separate identity • Unconditional acceptance • Help express needs, feelings • Assess and adjust to needs • Provide information • Provide experiences that diminish feelings of helplessness • Do not allow	• Continue assessment • Meet needs as they emerge • Understand reason for shifts in behaviour • Initiate rehabilitative plans • Reduce anxiety	
superficial: *Our telephone conversation focused on re-arranging another appointment and the patient sounded reluctant to discuss anything else* • *Actively avoids nurse/service provider: The patient did agree to schedule another appointment and this was done* *Service provider* • *No time for client meetings:Reluctant to commit to scheduling future appointments if the patient is unwilling to show up for these* • *Client meetings very short if they occur at all: Our telephone 'meetings' have tended to be short*	• Frequent changes of therapeutic approach • Sense of lack of connection • Increasing frustration • Length of meetings	• Respond to emergency • Practice non-directive listening • Focus client's energies • Clarify		

Table 4.2: continued/

Service provider

• Focus on instrumental tasks: *At the moment yes. The focus is on arranging meetings* • Decision that client is atypical of usual relationship: *No, this is quite common in some relationships* • Avoids client contact: *Reluctant to commit to scheduling future appointments if the patient is unwilling to show up for these*	vary • Place of meetings vary	preconceptions and expectations
	• Identify positive factors • Help plan for total needs • Facilitate forward movement of personality • Deal with therapeutic impasse	community agencies • Teach self-care • Terminate relationship

Note: Phases are overlapping

X				
MW	GR	O	WP	RP

Mark on the scale where check marks are concentrated within the table Checklists designed to assist in evaluating phase

Completed by Nurse Smith   Date: May 4th 2008

Table 4.3: Clinical example of Peplau's model at the relationship stage of orientation

Phases of the therapeutic relationship

	Mutual withdrawal	Grappling	Orientation	Working phase	Resolution phase
Client	• Forgets appointment/planned times: *The patient shows up for his scheduled appointment* • Cannot recall who nurse/service provider is: *Did not need reminding who I am or what my role is* • Unaware if nurse/service provider is available: *The patient remembered that he was supposed to meet with me and what mental health service I represented* • Content kept superficial: *No, content*	• Frequent changes of topics and approach: *Occasional change in topic, particularly when asked difficult questions* • Increasing frustration: *Frustration appears to be diminishing* • Sense of lack of connection:	• Seeks assistance: *Yes, has asked me to help him with his problem(s)* • Conveys educative needs: *Yes, the patient has stated that he wants to know more about what his problems are related to* • Asks questions: *Yes, occasionally and more often after a prompt* • Tests	• Identifies problems • Aware of time • Responds to help • Identifies with PP • Recognises and explores feelings • Fluctuates dependence, independence and interdependence in therapeutic relationship • Increases focal attention • Changes appearance (for better or worse) • Understands purpose of meeting • Maintains continuity between sessions (process and content) • Testing manoeuvres • Makes full use of services • Identifies new goals • Rapid shifts in behaviour; dependent–independent • Exploitative behaviour • Realistic exploitation • Self-directing • Develops skills in interpersonal relationships and problem solving • Displays changes in manner of	• Abandons old needs • Aspires to new goals • Becomes independent of helping person • Applies new problem-solving skills • Maintains changes in style of communication and interaction • Positive changes in view of self • Integrates illness • Exhibits ability to stand alone

Table 4.3: continued/

focused mainly on his problem(s) • Actively avoids nurse/service provider: No evidence of this	No evidence of this • Begins to dread meetings: No, patient appears to be interested in meeting – says he wants to address his problem(s)	parameters: Yes, occasionally • Shares preconceptions and expectations due to past experience: On occasion the patient will begin to open up and share; although this doesn't last for too long before he 'retreats' back into discussing safer subjects	decrease • Increase focal attention	communication (more open, flexible)	
Service provider					
• No time for client meetings:Not an issue, I have made time available • Client meetings very short if they occur at all: Meetings	• Frequent changes of therapeutic approach • Sense of lack of connection • Increasing frustration • Length of	• Respond to emergency: Not necessarily an emergency, but I have responded to the patients level of urgency for a meeting • Give parameters of meetings: Yes, we have explored the boundaries and limits of what I might be able to do • Explain roles: We have	• Maintain separate identity • Unconditional acceptance • Help express needs, feelings • Assess and adjust to needs • Provide information	• Continue assessment • Meet needs as they emerge • Understand reason for shifts in behaviour • Initiate rehabilitative plans	• Sustain relationship as long as patient feels necessary • Promote family interaction • Assist with goal setting • Teach

increasing in length and the patient is keeping his appointments

• Focus on instrumental tasks: *No, starting to examine his issues/problems*

• Decision that client is atypical of usual relationship: *No*

• Avoids client contact: *Not an issue, I have made time available*

meetings vary

• Place of meetings vary

examined the different types of help, and the different roles associated with this help, that I might offer

• Gather data: *Beginning to*

• Help client plan use of community resources and services: *Not yet, still working on identifying the nature of the problem(s)*

• Reduce anxiety and tension: *To some extent, although the patient still speaks of feeling tense and anxious on occasion*

• Practice non-directive listening: *Very much so*

• Focus client's energies: *Not yet*

• Clarify preconceptions and expectations: *This is in process, we are making some headway with this*

• Provide experiences that diminish feelings of helplessness

• Do not allow anxiety to overwhelm client

• Help focus on cues

• Help client develop responses to cues

• Use word stimuli

• Reduce anxiety

• Identify positive factors

• Help plan for total needs

• Facilitate forward movement of personality

• Deal with therapeutic impasse

preventive measures

• Utilise community agencies

• Teach self-care

• Terminate relationship

Note: Phases are overlapping

MW	GR	O	WP	RP
		X		

Mark on the scale where check marks are concentrated within the table

Checklists designed to assist in evaluating phase   Completed by Nurse Smith   Date: June 18th 2008

Table 4.4: Clinical example of Peplau's model at the relationship stage of working

Phases of the therapeutic relationship

Mutual withdrawal	Grappling	Orientation	Working phase	Resolution phase
Client				
• Forgets appointment/planned times: *The patient shows up for his scheduled appointment* • Cannot recall who nurse/service provider is: *Did not need reminding who I am or what my role is* • Unaware if nurse/service provider is available: *The patient remembered that he was supposed to meet with me and what mental*	• Frequent changes of topics and approach: *Occasional change in topic, particularly when asked difficult questions* • Increasing frustration: *Frustration appears to be diminishing* • Sense of lack of connection: *No evidence*	• Seeks assistance: *Yes, has asked me to help him with his problem(s)* • Conveys educative needs: *Yes, the patient has stated that he wants to know more about what his problems are related to* • Asks questions: *Yes, occasionally and more often after a prompt* • Tests parameters: *Yes,*	• Makes full use of services • Identifies new goals • Rapid shifts in behaviour; dependent—independent • Exploitative behaviour • Realistic exploitation • Self-directing • Develops skills in interpersonal relationships and problem solving • Displays changes in manner of communication • Identifies problems: *Yes, the patient says he feels insecure and threatened by the people in his local geographical area. This often results in his reluctance to go outside alone* • Aware of time: *Yes* • Responds to help: *Starting to, though he switches in and out of this willingness* • Identifies with PP: *?* • Recognises and explores feelings: *Starting to, though this is a work in progress* • Fluctuates dependence, independence and interdependence in therapeutic relationship: *Very much so* • Increases focal attention: *Yes, the patient's attention*	• Abandons old needs • Aspires to new goals • Becomes independent of helping person • Applies new problem-solving skills • Maintains changes in style of communication and interaction • Positive changes in view of self • Integrates illness • Exhibits ability to stand alone

				(more open, flexible)
health service I represented • Content kept superficial: No, content focused mainly on his problem(s) • Actively avoids nurse/service provider: No evidence of this	of this • Begins to dread meetings: No, patient appears to be interested in meeting – says he wants to address his problem(s)	occasionally • Shares preconceptions and expectations due to past experience: On occasion the patient will begin to open up and share; though this doesn't last for too long before he 'retreats' back into discussing safer subjects	is more and more directed towards his problem • Changes appearance (for better or worse): To some degree, appears to be starting to make more of an effort in self-grooming • Understands purpose of meeting: The patient says he does and appears to be engaging in some of the work • Maintains continuity between sessions (process and content): To some extent, though there is evidence of the usual 'ebb and flow' • Testing manoeuvres decrease: Yes, appears less suspicious and cautious of the health care staff now • Increase focal attention: To some extent, appears to be more focused on exploring the nature of his problem and exploring ways to address this	

Table 4.4: Continued/

Service provider

• No time for client meetings: *Not an issue, I have made time available* • Client meetings very short if they occur at all: *Meetings increasing in length and the patient is keeping his appointments* • Focus on instrumental tasks: *No, starting to examine his issues/ problems* • Decision that client is atypical of usual relationship: *No* • Avoids client contact: *Not an issue, I have made*	• Frequent changes of therapeutic approach • Sense of lack of connection • Increasing frustration • Length of meetings vary • Place of meetings vary	• Respond to emergency: *Not necessarily an emergency, but I have responded to the patients level of urgency for a meeting* • Give parameters of meetings: *Yes, we have explored the boundaries and limits of what I might be able to do* • Explain roles: *We have examined the different types of help, and the different roles associated with this help, that I might offer* • Gather data: *Beginning to* • Help client plan use of community resources and	• Maintain separate identity: *Yes, the patient does not appear to be triggering any significant transferential issues* • Unconditional acceptance: *Getting there, though this can be challenging at times* • Help express needs, feelings: *This is happening- there is evidence that the patient is expressing his feelings more* • Assess and adjust to needs: *Adjustment of my approach has occurred as a mechanism to encourage the patient to more freely express his emotions* • Provide information: *Frequently – for example, information provided about various mental health support facilities that are available in the patient's local area* • Provide experiences that diminish feelings of helplessness: *Very much so, helping the patient*	• Continue assessment • Meet needs as they emerge • Understand reason for shifts in behaviour • Initiate rehabilitative plans • Reduce anxiety • Identify positive factors • Help plan for total needs • Facilitate forward movement of personality	• Sustain relationship as long as patient feels necessary • Promote family interaction • Assist with goal setting • Teach preventive measures • Utilise community agencies • Teach self-care • Terminate relationship

time available

services: Not yet, still working on identifying the nature of the problem(s)
• Reduce anxiety and tension: To some extent, although the patient still speaks of feeling tense and anxious on occasion
• Practice non-directive listening: Very much so
• Focus client's energies: Not yet
• Clarify preconceptions and expectations: This is in process, we are making some headway with this

integrate new patterns about how powerful/powerless he feels in social situations where he feels threatened is a key element of our work
• Do not allow anxiety to overwhelm client: While the patient still reports occasional feelings of anxiety, there is no evidence that this has overwhelmed him
• Help focus on cues: Yes, we are examining the inter and intra-personal cues that appear to be linked to his specific feelings
• Help client develop responses to cues: Again yes, this is a key part of our ongoing work
• Use word stimuli: Sometimes

• Deal with therapeutic impasse

Note: Phases are overlapping

MW	GR	O	WP	RP
			x	

Completed by Nurse Smith   Date: July 20th 2008

Table 4.5: Clinical example of Peplau's model at the relationship stage of resolution

Phases of the therapeutic relationship

Mutual withdrawal	Grappling	Orientation	Working phase	Resolution phase
Client				
• Forgets appointment/ planned times: *The patient shows up for his scheduled appointment* • Cannot recall who nurse/service provider is: *Did not need reminding who I am or what my role is* • Unaware if nurse/service provider is available: *The patient remembered that he was supposed to meet with me and what mental*	• Frequent changes of topics and approach: *Occasional change in topic, particularly when asked difficult questions* • Increasing frustration: *Frustration appears to be diminishing* • Sense of lack of connection: *No evidence*	• Seeks assistance: *Yes, has asked me to help him with his problem(s)* • Conveys educative needs: *Yes, the patient has stated that he wants to know more about what his problems are related to* • Asks questions: *Yes, occasionally and more often after a prompt* • Tests parameters: *Yes,*	• Identifies problems: *Yes, patient says he feels insecure and threatened by the people in his local area. This often results in his reluctance to go outside alone* • Aware of time: *Yes* • Responds to help: *Starting to, though he switches in and out of this willingness* • Identifies with PP: *?* • Recognises and explores feelings: *Starting to, but this is work in progress* • Fluctuates dependence, independence and interdependence in therapeutic relationship: *Very much so* • Increases focal attention: *Yes, the patient's attention is more* • Makes full use of services: *Yes, appears to be engaged* • Identifies new goals: *Yes, patient has identified several new goals including finding part-time job* • Rapid shifts in behaviour; dependent– independent: *Some evidence of this, mostly showing independent behaviours* • Exploitative behaviour: *On occasion* • Realistic exploitation: *Yes, new goal of a part-time job*	• Abandons old needs: *Patient feels less need to isolate himself as a result of feeling afraid/ anxious* • Aspires to new goals: *Yes, wishes to work part-time and eventually full-time* • Becomes independent of helping person: *Getting there* • Applies new problem-solving skills: *Some evidence, e.g. figured out his transportation needs to be on*

health service / health care service provider represented
- Content kept superficial: *No, content focused mainly on his problem(s)*
- Actively avoids nurse/service provider: *No evidence of this*
- Begins to dread meetings: *No, patient appears to be interested in meeting – says he wants to address his problem(s)*

occasionally
- Shares preconceptions and expectations due to past experience: *On occasion the patient will begin to open up and share; though this doesn't last for too long before he 'retreats' back into discussing safer subjects*

and more directed towards his problem
- Changes appearance (for better or worse): *To some degree, starting to make more of an effort in self-grooming*
- Understands purpose of meeting: *Patient says he does and appears to be engaging in some of the work*
- Maintains continuity between sessions (process and content): *To some extent, though evidence of usual 'ebb and flow'*
- Testing manoeuvres decrease: *Yes, appears less suspiscious and cautious of the health care staff now*
- Increase focal attention: *To some extent, appears to be more focused on exploring the nature of his problem and exploring ways to address this*

is realistic
- Self-directing: *Certainly some evidence of this*
- Develops skills in interpersonal relationships and problem solving: *Evidence that patient is more comfortable in our interpersonal relationship, also willing to explore other new relationships*
- Displays changes in manner of communication (more open, flexible): *Patient displays far less evidence of being overly suspiscious and cautious of new relationships*

time for job
- Maintains changes in style of communication and interaction: *Evidence of change consistent over last 2 weeks*
- Positive changes in view of self: *Now says is able to cope with meeting new people in his job*
- Integrates illness
- Exhibits ability to stand alone: *Not only demonstrated this ability, now described as something to look forward to*

Table 4.5: Continued/

Service provider

• No time for client meetings: *Not an issue, I have made time available* • Client meetings very short if they occur at all: *Meetings increasing in length and the patient is keeping his appointments* • Focus on instrumental tasks: *No, starting to examine his issues/problems* • Decision that client is atypical of usual relationship: *No* • Avoids client	• Frequent changes of therapeutic approach • Sense of lack of connection • Increasing frustration • Length of meetings vary • Place of meetings vary	• Respond to emergency: *Not necessarily an emergency, but I have responded to the patients level of urgency for a meeting* • Give parameters of meetings: *Yes, we have explored the boundaries and limits of what I might be able to do* • Explain roles: *We have examined the different types of help, and the different roles associated with this help, that I might offer* • Gather data: *Beginning to* • Help client plan use of community resources and services: *Not yet, still*	• Maintain separate identity: *Yes, the patient does not appear to be triggering any significant transferential issues* • Unconditional acceptance: *Getting there, though this can be challenging at times* • Help express needs, feelings: *This is happening – there is evidence that the patient is expressing his feelings more* • Assess and adjust to needs: *Adjustment of my approach has occurred as a mechanism to encourage the patient to more freely express his emotions* • Provide information: *Frequently – for example, information provided about various mental health support facilities that are available in the patient's local area* • Provide experiences that diminish feelings of helplessness: *Very much so, helping the patient*	• Continue assessment • Meet needs as they emerge • Understand reason for shifts in behaviour • Initiate rehabilitative plans • Reduce anxiety • Identify positive factors • Help plan for total needs • Facilitate forward movement of personality	• Sustain relationship as long as patient feels necessary • Promote family interaction • Assist with goal setting • Teach preventive measures • Utilise community agencies • Teach self-care • Terminate relationship

contact: Not an issue, I have made time available

working on identifying the nature of the problem(s)
- Reduce anxiety and tension: *To some extent, although the patient still speaks of feeling tense and anxious on occasion*
- Practice non-directive listening: *Very much so*
- Focus client's energies: *Not yet*
- Clarify preconceptions and expectations: *This is in process, we are making some headway with this*

integrate new patterns about how powerful/powerless he feels in social situations where he feels threatened is a key element of our work
- Do not allow anxiety to overwhelm client: *While the patient still reports occasional feelings of anxiety, there is no evidence that this has overwhelmed him*
- Help focus on cues: *Yes, we are examining the inter and intra-personal cues that appear to be linked to his specific feelings*
- Help client develop responses to cues: *Again yes, this is akey part of our ongoing work*
- Use word stimuli: *Sometimes*

- Deal with therapeutic impasse

Note: Phases are overlapping

MW	GR	O	WP	RP
				x

Completed by Nurse Smith   Date: August 24th 2008

Morrison et al argue that it is necessary to undertake this exploratory study given that psychiatric nursing has changed during the past 30 years, yet Peplau's work roles for psychiatric nurses have remained largely unchanged. As a result of their findings, Morrison et al (1996) add the role of 'friend' to those identified by Peplau.

Forchuk et al (1998, 2000) report a research study that focused on bridging the transition from hospital, through discharge, to community. Using Peplau's model as the theoretical framework to guide this bridging process, the authors provide a very good example of how the model can be operationalised in clinical practice. It shows how there are a myriad of overlapping therapeutic relationships between patients and various mental healthcare workers, peers and family members. It provides data to show that the phases of the relationship can extend beyond the hospital setting and continue in the community. Further, Forchuk et al also illustrate how Peplau's different nursing roles are applied and situated within various stages of the hospital/community discharge process. An important finding from this paper is the reference to the overlapping therapeutic relationships that occur between patient and various mental healthcare workers and how these can facilitate the transition from hospital to community.

McNaughton (2005) reports on an attempt to apply Peplau's theory to the practice of home visiting. McNaughton purports that this was a naturalistic test drawing on five nurse–patient dyads who were obtained by means of purposeful sampling. Each of these dyads had experienced at least five visits (over varying lengths of time) and thus had a high chance of experiencing movement through Peplau's stages of the relationship. The study drew on Forchuk and Brown's (1989) instrument in order to measure the phase of the relationship; additional data from observation/field notes and audio recordings of the clinical visit were used to augment (triangulate) the instrument scores. Strong corroborating evidence for the scores recorded on the instrument were provided by the analysis of the audiotape transcripts. This paper, as a result, is a robust and fine example of how Peplau's model can be applied and used to underpin clinical nursing practice and that, despite some methodological problems, valid data can be obtained to demonstrate the application of Peplau's model. Not only do the findings in this paper support Peplau's central notion of progressing through stages of a therapeutic relationship, they also illustrate that Peplau's model is not restricted to psychiatric nursing settings.

Case studies

Lego (1998) draws on clinical examples as an attempt to apply Peplau's model to group psychotherapy. Lego's paper provides a solid example of some of Peplau's key ideas, perhaps most notably, the psychodynamic idea around previous experiences being transferred into the 'here and now'. It is not clear in the paper how Lego determines and/or explains when the relationship moves from one phase to the next, and she did not appear to say anything about Peplau's different nursing roles. So perhaps this is a good example of applying some of Peplau's ideas in clinical practice rather than a comprehensive application of her model.

Thelander (1997) attempts to apply Peplau's model to the treatment of people with so-called serious mental illness, and in so doing defends the application of Peplau in the field of psychiatric nursing. Drawing on his practice of psychotherapy, Thelander reflects on his practice of recent years and how Peplau's work has guided his practice; he then offers a case study. To his credit, he acknowledges that any 'outcomes' from this case study are anecdotal and are not rigorously tested. However, this is still valuable evidence. The strength of this paper resides in its attempt to apply Peplau's ideas about patterning, about earlier previous experiences being played out and subsequently challenged in the work with the psychiatric nurse in the 'here and now'. The authors of this book could see little evidence of Peplau's phases of the nurse–patient relationship. There is an abundance of evidence of working in the 'counsellor' role but little evidence of working in any other role. There does not appear to be any reference to moving through (or assessment of) the phases of the relationship which was somewhat surprising given that the case study describes a four and a half year study. The paper is arguably more about psychotherapy with patients with so-called 'mental illness' rather than the application of Peplau's model per se.

Usher and Arthur (1997) use a clinical situation rather than a person as a further example of applying Peplau to practice; this might even be thought of as a practice development paper. Usher and Arthur do refer to Peplau's different nursing roles and show how these are likely to be needed and utilised in their case example. They illustrate the operationalisation of the role of the teacher in the context of psychiatric nurses administering neuroleptic medication and educating the client about side-effects.

Price (1998) uses a case study to illustrate the application of Peplau's model to body image care. Price makes an interesting claim, namely that theory serves nursing practice in direct proportion to the extent to which it is accessible to patients, and thus evaluates how well Peplau's model serves nursing by means of its accessibility. Price's case study clearly shows a number of Peplau's key ideas, namely:

- The way nurses practice is closely bound to the development of their person.

- The meaning of the behaviour to the patient is the only relevant basis on which nurses can determine need.
- The nurse–patient relationship.
- The adoption of various nursing roles.
- The success of the therapeutic relationship is contingent upon nurses' understanding of themselves.

Price's paper also offers some interesting statements around trying to reconcile Peplau's model with a truncated duration for the nurse–patient relationship. Given Price's comments about the need for some haste (as a result of the limited time available), and Peplau's statements about the need for nurses to listen a lot and say very little, further work may be needed to reconcile these positions. Price concludes however that Peplau's model has sufficient clarity to be operationalised within body image nursing care.

Empirical papers that use Peplau's model as the theoretical underpinning

Beeber and Charlie (1998) undertook a study to examine reversal of symptoms of depression for women using a primary care health setting and used Peplau's model as their underpinning theoretical framework. Peden (1993) similarly focused on depressed women but sought to describe the process(es) of recovery in women who have been depressed. In addition to using Peplau's model as the underpinning theoretical framework, Peden also tried to use the model as a research method whereby she categorised/classified phenomena, sorted information about the phenomena and developed interventions.

Jacobson (1999) undertook a qualitative descriptive study to explore positive experiences of parenting and based this study on Peplau's model. Jacobson argues that the experiences and processes of positive parenting are very similar to some of Peplau's processes (or roles) of nursing: not least because they are both concerned with therapeutic relationships and communication. Jacobson concludes that these parallels merit further consideration. (Although it does strike the authors as being perhaps a little obvious that there are similarities between parenting and nursing given that the word nurse is derived from the old French word for nurturing a infant child. Also, both are concerned with nurturing the well-being and development of the other. However, we would concur that nurses could learn a lot about nursing from some parents and for that matter, some parents could learn a lot about parenting from some nurses.)

Suggested further reading: Theoretical comparisons and explorations of Peplau's model

- Forchuk (1991b): This paper gives a theoretical comparison to Orlando's (1961) nursing model that points out how Peplau's model did appear to emphasise longer-term nurse–patient relationships but that such relationships, and with that the individual stages, are flexible and amenable to being condensed.
- Martin et al (1992): This paper gives another theoretical comparison of Peplau's model, this time compared with the nursing models of Rogers (1970) and Parse (1981). These authors argue that nurses need to show how their practice is based on nursing science and on content that is relevant from other sciences and humanities.
- Forchuk and Dorsay (1995): This paper is an attempt to integrate Peplau's model with Wright and Leahey's (1984) family systems nursing theory. Forchuk and Dorsay argue that conceptual overlap does exist between the two models/theories, most especially in that both speak to a therapeutic process of engagement, phases of a relationship, interpersonal relations, patterns of relating, communication, and healing through personal growth.
- Reynolds (1997): This theoretical discussion paper focuses on three of Peplau's concepts (anxiety, self-esteem and hallucinations) and considers how they apply to practice.
- McCamant KL (2006): This is a theoretical comparison of Paterson and Zderads' (1988) humanistic nursing theory and Peplau's model. It concludes that Peplau's phases of the nurse–patient relationship are still applicable today, albeit dramatically truncated and abbreviated.
- Graham J (2006): This paper is another example of an attempt to compare nursing models/theories followed by a limited attempt at applying the model in practice, this time applying the model to the area/issue of caring for patients with end-stage kidney disease.

References

Aggleton P, Chalmers H (2000) *Nursing Models and Nursing Practice* 2nd edn. Macmillan Press, Basingstoke

Barker P (1998) The future of the Theory of Interpersonal relations? A personal reflection on Peplau's legacy. *Journal of Psychiatric and Mental Health Nursing* **5:** 213–20

Beeber LS, Bourbonniere M (1998) The concept of interpersonal pattern in Peplau's Theory of Nursing. *Journal of Psychiatric and Mental Health Nursing* **5:** 187–92

Beeber LS, Charlie ML (1998) Depressive symptom reversal for women in a primary care setting: A pilot study. *Archives of Psychiatric Nursing* **12**(5): 247–54

Benner P (1984) *From Novice to Expert: Excellence and Power in Clinical Practice*. Addison-Wesley, New York

Cutcliffe JR (2004) *The Inspiration of Hope in Bereavement Counselling*. Jessica Kingsley, London

Cutcliffe J, Wieck L (2008) Salvation or damnation: Deconstructing nursing's aspirations to professional status. *Journal of Nursing Management* **16**: 499–507

Dewey J (2007) John Dewey: Philosophy of Education. Available from: http:// wilderdom.com/experiential/JohnDeweyPhilosophyEducation.html [accessed 2007]

Forchuk C (1991a) Peplau's Theory: Concepts and their relations. *Nursing Science Quarterly* **4**(2): 54–60

Forchuk C (1991b) A comparison of the works of Peplau and Orlando. *Archives of Psychiatric Nursing* **5**(1): 38–45

Forchuk C, Brown B (1989) Establishing a nurse client relationship. *Journal of Psychosocial Nursing* **27**(2): 30–4

Forchuk C, Dorsay JP (1995) Hildegard Peplau meets family systems nursing: Innovation in theory-based practice. *Journal of Advanced Nursing* **21**: 110–115

Forchuk C, Jewell J, Schofield R, Sircelj M, Valledor T (1998) From hospital to community: Bridging therapeutic relationships. *Journal of Psychiatric and Mental Health Nursing* **5**: 197–202

Forchuk C, Schofield R, Martin ML, Sircelj M, Woodcox V, Jewell J, Valledor T, Overby B, Chan L (2000) Bridging the discharge process: staff and client experiences over time. *Journal of American Psychiatric Nurses Association* **4**(4): 128–33

Freud S (1936) *The Problem with Anxiety*. WW Norton, New York

Graham J (2006) Nursing theory and clinical practice: How three nursing models can be incorporated into the care of patients with end stage kidney disease. *The Canadian Association of Nephrology Nurses and Technologists Journal* **16**(4): 28–31

Haber J (2000) Hildegard E. Peplau: The psychiatric nursing legacy of a legend. *Journal of the American Psychiatric Nurses Association* **6**(2): 56–62

Jacobson GJ (1999) Parenting processes: A descriptive exploratory study using Peplau's Theory. *Nursing Science Quarterly* **12**(3): 240–4

Kuhn T (1962) *The Structure of Scientific Revolutions*. 3rd edn. Chicago University Press, Chicago

Lego S (1998) The application of Peplau's theory to group psychotherapy. *Journal of Psychiatric and Mental Health Nursing* **5**: 193–6

McCamant KL (2006) Humanistic nursing, Interpersonal Relations Theory, and the empathy-altruism hypothesis. *Nursing Science Quarterly* **19**(4): 334–8

McNaughton DB (2005) A Naturalistic test of Peplau's Theory in home visiting. *Public Health Nursing* **22**(5): 429–38

Martin M, Forchuk C, Santopinto M, Butcher HK (1992) Alternative approaches to nursing practice: Application of Peplau, Rogers and Parse. *Nursing Science Quarterly* **5**(2): 80–5

Maslow A (1954) *Motivation and Personality*. Harper Row, New York

Morrison EG, Shealy AH, Kowalski C, LaMont J, Range BA (1996) Work roles of Staff Nurses in Psychiatric settings. *Nursing Science Quarterly* **9**(1): 17–21

Orlando IJ (1961) *The Dynamic Nurse–Patient Relationship: Function, Process and Principles*. Putnam, New York

Parse RR (1981) *Man-Living-Health: A Theory of Nursing*. John Wiley & Sons, New York

Paterson JG, Zderad LT (1988) *Humanistic Nursing*. National League for Nursing Press, New York (Originally published 1976)

Pearson A, Vaughan B (1986) *Nursing Models for Practice*. Heinemann, Oxford

Peden AR (1993) Recovering in depressed women: Research with Peplau's Theory. *Nursing Science Quarterly* **6**(3): 140–6

Peplau HE (1987) Interpersonal constructs in nursing practice. *Nurse Education Today* **7**(5): 201–8

Peplau HE (1988) *Interpersonal Relations in Nursing: A Conceptual Frame of Reference for Psychodynamic Nursing*. 2nd edn. Macmillan Press, Houndmills, Basingstoke

Peplau HE (1991) Interpersonal relations: A theoretical framework for application in nursing practice. *Nursing Science Quarterly* **5**(1): 13–8

Peplau HE (1995) *Schizophrenia – Conference Presentation*. Annual Conference, University of Ulster, Northern Ireland

Peplau HE (1997) Peplau's Theory of Interpersonal Relations. *Nursing Science Quarterly* **10**(4): 162–7

Price B (1998) Explorations in body image care: Peplau and practice knowledge. *Journal of Psychiatric and Mental Health Nursing* **5**: 179–86

Rawlins RP, Williams SR, Beck CK (1993) *Mental Health – Psychiatric Nursing: A Holistic Life-Cycle Approach*. Mosby, New York

Reynolds WJ (1997) Peplau's Theory in practice. *Nursing Science Quarterly* **10**(4): 168–70

Riehl JP, Roy C (1980) *Conceptual Models for Nursing Practice*. Appleton-Century-Crofts, New York

Rogers ME (1970) *An Introduction to the Theoretical Basis of Nursing*. Davis, Philadelphia

Schneider JK, Hornberger S, Booker J, Davis A, Kralicek R (1993) A medication discharge planning program: Measuring the effects on re-admissions. *Clinical Nursing Research* **2**(1): 41–53

Sofarelli M, Brown R (1998) The need for nursing leadership in uncertain times. *Journal of Nursing Management* **6**(4): 201–7

Stenberg College (2007). http://www.stenbergcollege.com/rpn.html [accessed 2007]

Sullivan HS (1952) *The Interpersonal Theory of Psychiatry*. Norton, New York

Sullivan HS (1953) *Conceptions of Modern Psychiatry*. Norton, New York

Sullivan EJ, Decker PJ (2001) *Effective Leadership and Management in Nursing* 5th edn. Upper Saddle River, NJ: Prentice Hall

Suppe F, Jacox A (1985) Philosophy of science and the development of nursing theory. *Annual Review of Nursing Research* **3**: 241–67

Thelander BL (1997) The psychotherapy of Hildegard Peplau in the treatment of people with serious mental illness. *Perspectives in Psychiatric Care* **33**(3): 24–9

Thompson IE, Melia KM, Boyd KM (2000) *Nursing Ethics* (4th Edn). Churchill Livingstone, Edinburgh

Usher KJ, Arthur D (1997) Nurses and neuroleptic medication: Applying theory to a working relationship with clients and their families. *Journal of Psychiatric and Mental Health Nursing* **4**: 117–23

Varcarolis EM, Carson VB, Shoemaker NC (2006) *Foundations of Psychiatric Mental Health Nursing: A Clinical Approach*. WB Saunders, St Louis

Wright LM, Leahey M (1984) *Nurses and Families: A Guide to Family Assessment and Intervention*. FA Davis Co, Philadelphia

CHAPTER 5

Imogene King's Conceptual System and Theory of Goal Attainment

Introduction

When approaching the work of Imogene King (1981, 1997, 2001), it is helpful to recognise that it is comprised of a conceptual framework, a theory of goal attainment and a model of nurse–patient transactions. King began to conceive a frame of reference for nursing in the 1960s while she was an associate professor of nursing developing a new graduate degree programme at Loyola University in Chicago (see King, 1971: 2, Gulitz and King, 1988). She sought to identify essential components of nursing that had persisted over time (King, 1971). She believed that this would help teachers to identify and select the relevant concepts central to nursing practice to teach their nursing students.

King formulated and published her Conceptual Framework in the book *Toward a Theory for Nursing* in 1971. It was her belief that the theoretical frame of reference she presented had been derived from the basic elements that had and would continue to persist over time in nursing (King, 1971: 120). She acknowledged that the conceptual frame of reference was abstract and dealt with only a few elements of concrete situations. However, she believed that the framework served three purposes: it provided a way of thinking about the real world of nursing; it suggested an approach for selecting concepts perceived to be fundamental for the practice of professional nursing; and it showed a process for developing concepts that symbolised experiences within the physical, psychological and social environment of nursing.

In 1981, King published a second book entitled *A Theory for Nursing: Systems, Concepts, Process*, which presented a refinement of the Conceptual Framework (King, 1981:10–12), definitions of several key concepts and an introduction to the Theory of Goal Attainment (King, 1981: 141–150). The theory describes the nature of nurse–client interactions that lead to achievement of goals. This book also contains suggestions for recording nursing care within a goal-oriented nursing record (King, 1981: 164–177).

The model has remained essentially unchanged since publication of the 1981 book. However, King worked continuously, even well past retirement, writing about and presenting her work, while also educating and mentoring nurses interested in furthering her work. She has been acknowledged as a generous mentor who was able to 'relinquish the extension of ideas and ideals to which she was committed' and supported a new generation of theorists (Frey and Sieloff, 1995). She contributed to *Advancing King's Systems Framework and Theory of Nursing* which was published in 1995 as a compilation of the work of nurses who had been extending and expanding her work. Sieloff and Frey have edited a recently published book entitled *Middle Range Theory Development Using King's Conceptual System* (2007). This book describes the continuous development and testing of middle range theories applied to individuals, groups, families and organisations using King's life work.

In 1997, Imogene King wrote a review of her Conceptual System and her Theory of Goal Attainment. Near the end of that article, she reflected on over 50 years of nursing work and shared an unpublished definition which she had written some 15 years prior:

King's law of nurse–patient interaction: 'Nurses and patients in mutual presence, interacting purposefully, make transactions in nursing situations based on each individual's perceptions, purposeful communication and valued goals.'

(King, 1997a)

While her work is generally known to be based on systems theory, she also clearly places an emphasis on interaction theory. As such, her framework has proven to be particularly useful for nurses whose social interactions with patients are a key focus of their practice. Also, since the Theory of Goal Attainment is not applied directly to practice but through nurses' understanding of concepts and through critical thinking, it can be applied broadly to almost any nursing situation. In fact, King believes that many nurses use the Theory of Goal Attainment when interacting professionally with patients although they may not recognise it as such (King, 1981: 157).

The literature is full of examples of applications of King's open systems model in many different situations. Frey et al. (2002: 109) listed all the knowledge building practice and research publications using King's Conceptual System and/or Theory of Goal Attainment between the years 1973 and 2000. The total number adds up to 574 different types of publications and topics. Gulitz and King (1988), for example, demonstrated the application of the model to curriculum development. Frey et al. (1995) compared and contrasted the cultural relevance of the Conceptual Framework in Japan, Sweden and the United States, while Husting (1997) provided a transcultural critique of the theory. King (2006) described the application to nursing administration. Khowaja (2006) and Fewster-Thuente and Velsor-Friedrich (2008) wrote of its utility for interdisciplinary collaboration. Messmer (2006) has illustrated the relevance of King's theory as a professional practice model for Magnet organisations. Most recently, Killeen and King (2007) have written about the usefulness of the Conceptual Systems as a structure in technology use for nursing informatics.

According to King (1981, see also Fawcett, 2001) the framework and the theory contain multiple, carefully defined concepts that can be used to develop theories, and, in fact, Fawcett (2001: 313) cited a number of examples of published theories based on her work as of 2001: theory of families, children and chronic illness; theory of departmental power that has been developed from the concept of 'power'; theory related to patient satisfaction that has been developed from the concept of 'perception'; theories of family health and theory of interpersonal perceptual awareness. Previously, King had also noted that instruments had been developed to measure the concepts of her framework (King, 1997a). For example, the Sieloff-King Assessment of Departmental Power (SKADP) and its revision (SKAGPO) (Sieloff, 2003) and the Assessment of Functional Abilities and Goal Attainment Scale (King, 2003) are representative of valid and reliable instruments that can be used in nursing research to test hypotheses generated from her work.

The conceptual framework that King developed involves three interacting sets of systems. The innermost systems are the personal systems which are comprised of individuals. King describes humans as open systems interacting with the environment. Man, the human organism, is the central focus for the framework (King, 1971). When individuals interact, they form interpersonal systems. These can be as small as a dyad such as a nurse and a patient or a larger group, such as a family. The outermost systems are social systems. These are the largest systems and are defined by King (1981: 119) as 'composed of human beings with prescribed roles and positions who use resources to accomplish personal and organisational goals'. Examples of social systems include religious and educational organisations, hospitals and employers (King, 1981: 11-12) (*Figure 5.1*).

The Theory of Goal Attainment exists in the context of this conceptual framework. The theory describes the nature of the nurse–client interaction that leads to the achievement of goals as follows. The nurse and the patient work together to define and set goals. They both interact with each other and react to each other. At the end of this process, if they have set a goal, a transaction has occurred. The nurse and patient also mutually decide on a way to achieve the goal and create a plan of action(s). Transactions occur related to the health of the patient, and the plan for meeting the goals may involve interactions with other systems, such as other healthcare workers,

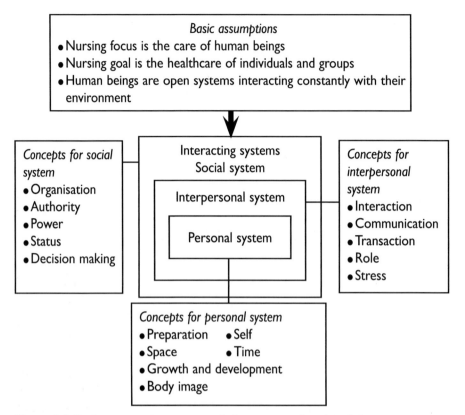

Figure 5.1. Basic assumptions, personal , interpersonal and social systems.

the patient's family, or larger systems. (King, 1981: 141–161; 1991; 1995: 25–32) (see *Box 5.1*).

After the transaction has occurred, there remains the critical component of documentation. The nurse documents the goal(s) which has been agreed upon. This not only facilitates communication with other nurses and healthcare workers but it also helps to provide a way to determine whether or not the goal is achieved (see King, 1981: 149). The assessment is important to King's goal attainment theory and the emphasis on outcomes makes the theory particularly relevant in today's quality-driven healthcare environment (King, 2007). Messmer (2006) discusses King's theory in the context of Magnet organisations and the centrality of empirical outcomes in the new Magnet model (American Nurses Credentialing Center, 2008), which underscores the importance of connecting care to consumer outcomes.

It is possible to argue that the inclusion of concepts such as self, human interactions, and perception supports the holistic approach through the framework to practice. However, another perspective can also be argued. King's framework describes environments within which human beings

---

Box 5.1: Propositions of the Theory of Goal Attainment

- If perceptual accuracy is present in nurse–client interactions, transactions will occur
- If nurse and client make transactions, goals will be attained
- If goals are attained, satisfactions will occur
- If goals are attained, effective nursing care will occur
- If transactions are made in nurse–client interactions, growth and development will be enhanced
- If role expectations and role performance as perceived by nurse and client are congruent, transactions will occur
- If role conflict is experienced by nurse or client or both, stress in nurse–client interactions will occur
- If nurses with special knowledge and skills communicate appropriate information to clients, mutual goal setting and goal attainment will occur

(King, 1981: 149)

---

exist and the concepts in this framework are the organising dimensions that represent the knowledge essential for understanding the interactions among the three systems (King, 1995b:18) The perspective in the framework, from the individual system to examine the role it plays in the larger systems describes a functionalist, rather than a holistic, approach. This is not to say that the perspective is not valid, but simply that it cannot be contrasted to a mechanical or reductionist perspective as 'more holistic'.

Over the years, there have been criticisms of Imogene King's Conceptual System. She wrote extensively in defence of her work and published many articles which explained or expanded upon her original writings. In 1994, Carter and Dufour wrote a critique of the critiques relative to King's theory. They summarised the most common criticisms which include: the limitation to societies with Western cultural sick role attitudes (see also Meleis, 1991; Meleis and Jones, 1983); the questionable applicability to those who cannot interact competently with the nurse (see, for example, Ackermann et al., 1989); and the lack of specific definitions and guidelines to direct the nursing process (Fawcett, 1989).

Nursing

Long before the birth of the information age and the evolution of technological complexity in healthcare, King understood that there were both eternal elements of nursing as well as transitory and changeable elements. She expressed a personal concern about the changes influencing nursing, a conscious awareness of the knowledge explosion and an interest in the essential components of nursing (King, 1971: 2). She found that several thoughts were consistently expressed: nursing is complex because of the human variables in nursing situations; nurses play many roles in social institutions; and the past and present influence the responsibilities and decisions made by nurses. King (1971: 19) first undertook her work of developing a conceptual framework by asking several questions:

- What are some of the social and educational changes in the United States that have influenced changes in nursing?
- What basic elements are continuous throughout these changes in nursing?
- What is the scope of the practice of nursing, and in what kinds of setting do nurses perform their functions?
- Are the current goals of nursing similar to those of the past half century?
- What are the dimensions of practice that have given the field of nursing a unifying focus over time?

The questions established a framework for her thinking and further prompted the exploration of the field of systems analysis, general systems theory, and also the identification of concept synthesis into a conceptual framework through another set of questions (King, 1971:19–20):

- What kinds of decisions are nurses required to make in the course of their roles and responsibilities?
- What kind of information is essential for them to make decisions?
- What are the alternatives in nursing situations?
- What alternative courses of actions do nurses have in making critical decisions about another individual's care, recovery and health?
- What skills do nurses now perform and what knowledge is essential for nurses to make decisions about alternatives?

King defined nursing as: 'a process of action, reaction, and interaction whereby nurse and client share information about their perceptions in the nursing situation' (King, 1971: 25). She described the goal of nursing as bringing a person closer to a healthy state (King, 1997a; 2001) and to help individuals to attain, maintain and restore their health so that they can function in their roles (King, 1981: 3–4, 13). According to King, if this was not possible, then nurse(s) help individuals die with dignity (King, 1981: 13). King has emphasised that the means to attain goals at each level of the three dynamic interacting systems (i.e. personal, interpersonal and social) are different (King, 1995a: 24). She observed that 'nurses are the key persons in the healthcare system who identify the goals and the means to help individuals and families attain goals' (King, 1995a: 24).

She acknowledged outcomes as satisfaction with performing activities of daily living, success in performing activities in one's usual role and achievement of immediate and long-range goals (King, 1981: 1). She further acknowledged that nurse(s) use knowledge and skills to help individuals and groups cope with existing problems and learning ways of adjusting changes in daily activities (King, 1981: 3). The functions of nursing include strategies such as teaching, supporting, counselling, guiding and motivating. Nurses integrate knowledge from the natural and behavioural sciences and humanities and apply it in concrete situations so that they can function in their roles and meet the goal of health for individuals and groups under normal and stressful conditions (King, 1981: 8). Techniques used by nurses include: assessment, communication, systematic gathering of information, interviews, measurement and observation.

King has called 'a nursing act' the basic unit of nursing behaviour and she has identified the components of nursing process as: action, reaction, interaction, and transaction (King, 1981: 2). The nurse–patient transaction model is comprised of a process of mutual perception, judgement and action. The actions lead to reaction, interaction and transaction. Although depicted in a linear model, there is constant feedback within the cycle and the process is dynamic.

The nursing process entails essential functions of nurses such as assessment of the patient's health, formulation of a plan on the basis of the information gathered, implementation of a plan of action and evaluation of its effectiveness (King, 1981: 9). Skills of observation and measurement are important in this process as are critical thinking skills (King, 1981: 9).

Health

Health is a dynamic ever-changing process that is a state of being. It is non-linear and fluid throughout the life cycle. Health is a functional state and illness represents interference in that functional state. In 1990, King published an article that discussed the meaning of health and its relevance for nursing science. This article was both a synthesis of literature and a concept presentation (King, 1990).

Her literature review is interesting, as it showed common characteristics of health cited by many authors. These included that health is genetic, relative, subjective, dynamic, environmental, functional, cultural and perceptual (King, 1990: 125). Health can be viewed as a state, a process, a diagnosis, a task, a response or a goal. The synthesis showed that health concerns the whole person interacting with the environment (see also King, 1971: 24).

The person constantly adapts to meet the needs of both the internal and external environments. The internal environment is comprised of such things as the organs, cells, hormones, and inner thoughts while the external environment is comprised of such things as sound, air, pollution, and food. In King's definition: 'health is a dynamic state in the life cycle of a person which implies adjustment to stressors in the internal and external environment through optimum use of resources to achieve maximum potential for daily living' (King, 1971: 24).

King (1981: 4–5) has also stated that health is a process of human growth and development. It relates to the way individuals deal with the stress of growth and development while functioning within the cultural pattern in which they were born and to which they attempt to conform/adjust. Health is necessary to lead a useful, satisfying, productive and happy life (King, 1981: 4) and it is viewed as the ability to function in daily life and in social roles. King's definition regarding health has been criticised in the literature (e.g. Fawcett, 1984) as limiting. However, for King, when factors arise that interfere with the performance of daily activities and maintenance of independence, it is important to identify measurable indicators (King, 1981: 5–6). And, because the concept of health is complicated and multidimensional, relative and subjective, in the context of a complex environment, measures of health present a challenge. Her definition can be viewed as a response to that challenge.

With her Conceptual Framework and interrelated concepts, she presents one way of identifying the health needs, where health is a function of persons interacting with the environment (King, 1981: 7–8). Within the Theory of Goal Attainment, she provides a structure within which to document nursing care and achievement of goal(s). The findings/observations can then be used to demonstrate the effectiveness of nursing care by using both quantitative and qualitative evaluation methods relative to health as the goal of nursing.

Interestingly, in 1995, Cynthia Kelsey Winker reflected on King's 1971 definition in which she wrote that health encompasses the whole man. She proposed a new definition consistent with a holistic rather than mechanistic perspective such that health is the ability of the individual to create meaningful symbols based on either biological or human values within his or her own cultural and individual values systems.

Persons

According to King (1981: 10), the person is a unique total system (i.e. personal system) that is dynamic in its continuous interaction with the environment and whose perceptions influence its interactions and its health. Originally, King (1981: 10, 19–20) made nine assumptions about the person. She described person(s) as: social, sentient, rational, reacting, perceiving, controlling, purposeful, action-oriented, and time-oriented. Although there have been no major changes to the framework or the Theory of Goal Attainment since the 1981 textbook, King has provided explanations, clarifications and expansions of the concepts through numerous publications. The changes include, for example, addition of the word 'spiritual' to the assumptions about human beings and definitions of such concepts as learning and coping (King, 2001). Interestingly, many of the changes, additions and clarifications are related to the concept person. King (1981: 19–20) has presented three basic premises about the person as follows: human beings/persons are reactive beings, time-oriented and social. In 1981, she also stated that, 'Through language human beings have found a symbolic way of communicating thoughts, actions, customs, and beliefs. Persons exhibit common characteristics such as the ability to perceive, to think, to feel, to choose between alternative courses of action, to set goals, to select the means to achieve the goals, and to make decisions.' These characteristics indicated to King that human beings are reacting beings (King 1981: 19).

King (1981: 19–47) has proposed six relevant concepts for nurses to understand the person as an open system: perception, self, growth and development, body image, time, and space. She has defined these concepts carefully followed with examples/applications in her book on systems, concepts and processes. Perception is described as a process of human transactions with the environment; it gives meaning to one's experience, represents one's image of reality and influences one's behaviour. The perception of one's health may be different from the signs and symptoms one's behaviour manifests to others. Self is the composite of thoughts and feelings which constitute a person's awareness of individual existence. The self is reflected in patterns of growth and development and in the structure and function of the human being. Growth and development are a function of genetic endowment, meaningful and satisfying experiences, and an environment conducive to helping individuals move towards maturity. Body image, both conscious and unconscious, is the person's perception of his or her own body, other's reactions to his or her appearance and is a result of others' reactions to self. Space is universal in that it exists everywhere. It is subjective, though, because perception of space is often rooted in culture. It is also influenced by individual needs and past experiences. It is situational in that some situations pull people together while others push them apart. Use of and defence of space are nonverbal communications. Time is a sequence of events moving onwards to the future and influenced by the past. It is a term used to give order to events and to determine duration between one event and another as experienced by each human being.

King (1981: 8) also stated that the person has three fundamental health needs: the need for health information that is useable when it is needed; care that seeks to prevent illness; and care when unable to care for themselves. In 1995 (1995b: 18), she stated that the unit of analysis in this framework is human behaviour in a variety of social environments and the need (any or all of the three) of each individual depends on the characteristics of that individual and how he or she is relating to the environment.

Environment

According to King (1981: 10–13), persons are open systems that are in constant interaction with their environment through three interacting systems. These are the personal system, the interpersonal system, and the social system. Since King considers the individual human being to be one type of system. The discussion of personal system or environment has been presented under the section 'Persons'.

King (1981: 141) has described and defined the three interacting systems as:

Individuals comprise one type of system in the environment called personal systems. Individuals interact to form dyads, triads, and small and large groups, which comprise another type of system called interpersonal systems. Groups with special interests and needs form organisations, which make up communities and societies and are called social systems.

The framework that is comprised of the three systems describes environments within which human beings grow, develop and perform daily activities. The concepts represent knowledge essential for understanding the interactions between the three systems (King, 1995b: 18).

Interpersonal systems

Interpersonal systems occur when humans socialise (King, 1981: 10–11). Selected concepts that help nurses to understand interactions of human beings are interaction, communication, transaction, role, stress, and coping. These concepts are carefully defined and described with examples/implications for nursing in King's book (1981: 59–103). According to King, interaction is the verbal and nonverbal behaviour between the individual and the environment or between two or more individuals. Communication means the transmission of information directly between persons, or indirectly through some media such as by telephone or email. Transaction is the interaction between a person and another person or a person and the environment for the purpose of goal attainment. Role is described as the expected behaviour of a person in a specific position and the rules that direct the interactions between two or more persons. Stress means the exchange of energy that is either positive or negative between a person and the environment. Objects, events and persons can all serve as stressors. Interestingly, coping was considered important by King but this concept has not been defined in her book.

Social systems

Social systems occur when interpersonal systems come together to form larger systems such as religious organisations, schools, and corporations (King, 1981: 11).

According to King (1981: 12) the concepts that provide knowledge for nurses and help them to function in healthcare systems are social roles, authority, power, status and decision making. These concepts are defined and described with examples/implications for nursing in King's book (1981: 113–135). Role is described as a set of behaviours adopted when occupying a position in a social system (King, 1981:93). Authority is defined as a transactional process characterised by active, reciprocal relations in which members' values, backgrounds and perceptions play a role in defining, validating and accepting the [directions] of individuals within an organisation (King, 1981: 124). Power has been described as 'the capacity to use resources in organisations to achieve goals; process whereby one or more persons influence other persons in a situation and capacity or ability of a group to achieve goals' (King, 1981: 124). Status is the position of an individual in a group or a group in relation to other groups in an organisation (King, 1981: 129). Decision making has been defined as a 'dynamic and systemic process by which a goal-directed choice of perceived alternatives is made, and acted upon, by individuals or groups to answer and attain goals (King, 1981: 132).

As is the case with personal systems, both interpersonal and social systems are open systems and are, therefore, sensitive to environmental changes. A change in the environment can have a profound impact on any open system. The overall health of a system is strongly linked with its ability to anticipate and adapt to environmental change. Similarly, the health of the environment is interconnected with the transactions taking place in the personal, interpersonal and social systems and all subsystems operating within them (see Walonick, 1993).

Clinical application

Anna is a 12-year-old girl who has cystic fibrosis (CF), which was diagnosed when she was 5 years old. CF is an inherited (genetic) disease characterised by abnormal secretion of the exocrine glands. It is the most common lethal genetic disease among Caucasian Americans affecting about 1 in 2400 live births. Although it can involve many organs, CF particular affects the lungs, digestive system, sweat glands, and male/female fertility. Due to the failure of the functioning of the chlorine channel, CF causes thick, sticky mucus to build up in and prevent proper functioning of the organs. Diabetes mellitus (type 1 or 2) may be present. Close attention to and prompt treatment of respiratory and digestive complications have dramatically increased the expected lifespan of a person with CF (Black et al., 2001; LeMone and Bruke, 2004; Hockenberry et al., 2003).

Anna's CF has been very mild and the illness has had only a minor impact on her health. She lives with her father Jack, mother Ellie and a younger sister Alice in a small rural town. The air quality is very good (there is no industrial pollution), the humidity is generally 60–70% during the summer and the temperature is reasonably mild during the winter. Anna's father used to smoke a pipe, but he quit smoking soon after his daughter was born. The home has been smoke-free for almost 12 years. Genetic testing has shown that the younger sibling, Alice, does not carry the gene defect.

Anna had not been in school for two days, since she had mild cold symptoms with coughing. Over the weekend, Anna was admitted to the paediatric ward of a local hospital after presenting in the emergency room with the cold symptoms and a mildly elevated temperature (36.8^0 C). A chest x-ray has been taken to rule out bronchopneumonia/infection and prophylactic (oral) antibiotics have been started. Anna has been almost symptom-free all her life due to careful attention to her life-style at home (i.e. balanced meals; high-protein, high-calorie, high-salt, low-fat diet; vitamin and mineral supplements including fat-soluble vitamins) and school (i.e. yearly influenza vaccine, avoiding exposure to large crowds and infected people).

The initial action of her primary nurse on the ward was to record biographicl data, and to interact with Anna and mother Ellie to obtain more information about the activities of daily living (ADL). The nurse collected the information shown in *Tables 5.1 and 5.2* during discussion with Anna and her mother. In the following example, nursing aims at restoring and maintaining those aspects of Anna's life, which she and her mother are concerned about and which affect Anna's health.

When the nurse applies King's framework, assessment is composed of perception and action, and problems are identified through reaction and interaction. Transaction leads to the formulation of a care plan and its implementation. The care plan is a statement agreed upon by the nurse, Anna and her family members. The care plan is a guide to the nature of the interactive process to be engaged in while nursing takes place. It is a description for action, a means by which to judge the reactions and an account of planned interaction. Once the transaction has been agreed upon, specific goals are set in order to give direction and to be used to determine (evaluate) the reaction. In Anna's case the nurse was able to identify problems in the performance of the activities of daily living related to this girl's social systems network, perception, interpersonal relationships and health. The goals were written by the nurse together with Anna and her mother Ellie. Since her father Jack was at home with Anna's little sister Alice, it was agreed that the care plan would be re-visited and re-assessed together with him at the earliest convenience (*Table 5.3*)

When the nurse was talking with Anna and Ellie, she perceived that they were a well-groomed daughter and mother who appeared to be comfortable in the examination room and who made eye contact with the nurse. Anna looked slim, but her physical development/appearance was normal, and comparable for her age. When Anna was talking with the nurse about her cough and the CF, her perception regarding her body image seemed realistic. As they interacted, the nurse found out that Anna is very intelligent and excels at school (growth and development). Anna views herself as essentially moderately healthy (self), but she also seems to understand that CF is a chronic condition. Anna's mother Ellie (38 years) is an elementary school teacher and she has just recently started to work half-time at the local school. Anna's father Jack (40 years) is an engineer and has to travel several days per month for business. The mother's half-time job and father's occasional absence from home have been a little stressful for the family, but also exciting because during the afternoons, Anna takes care of her sister

Table 5.1. Example of biographical information
Name: Anna Elisabeth Jones Age: 12 years   Date of birth: May 17, xxxx Prefers to be addressed: Anna
Mother and father: Ellie and Jack Jones Mother's profession: School teacher Father's profession: Engineer Siblings: Alice Jones (younger sister) Address: 22 Blackberry Road, xx, xx Tel: xx - 831-198
Weight: 28 kg (60 lb)   Height: 138 cm (54") Temp: 36.8⁰C   Pulse: 100/min   BP: 116/75mmHg   Resp: 90/min Chest x-ray: no new pathological findings Pulse oximetry, oxygen saturation (SaO_2) >95%, $PaCO_2$ <42mmHg B-glucose: 180 g/mol (normal) Haemoglobin (Hgb), hematocrit (Hct) and White blood cell count (WBC): normal

Table 5.2. Collecting information about the activities of daily living

ADL	Social Systems	Perceptions	Interpersonal relations	Health state/assessment
Breathing	• Coughing: some mucus production • Embarrassed when she has symptoms of her CF in front of friends	'My cough started to get bad at school. When the coughing starts, I can't stop it.'	Conscious that noisy, continuous coughing is distracting the class and is uncomfortable having to use tissues for the mucus	Coughing up some mucus Chest X –ray: no new pathological findings
Eating and drinking	• Mother prepares nutritious meals every day – normal/decreased appetite	'I don't always like vegetables, but I love spaghetti and ice-cream. My mom thinks that I'm skinny'	'My mom cooks every day good and healthy food for all of us and we eat our dinner together every evening'	Underweight, pale (blood glucose: normal) Well hydrated (pre-requisite for productive coughing)
Eliminating	• Independent: no problems with bowel or urinating	'I want to go in the bathroom alone, not with mom or Alice'	Embarrassed by need to discuss elimination	Opens bowels daily Does not need to urinate at night
Movement and posture	• Restricted in attending sport activities at school (some visible 'barrel-chest' and 'clubbed fingers)	'I cannot run or play as much as the other kids, because then my breathing gets hard'	Slightly isolated at school when other kids attend sport activities	Can walk around the unit and get to the cafeteria without getting breathless
Sleep and rest	• Likes to sleep in own bedroom at home • Has been waking 1–2 times/night because of the coughing	'I haven't been able to sleep well: I start coughing during the night. Then I'm tired all day'	'I don't want to wake up my family during the night when I start coughing'	Bed at 8:30 pm, up at 7:30 am. Has been napping during the afternoon

Table 5.2/continued

ADL	Social systems	Perceptions	Interpersonal relations	Health state/assessment
Dress and undress	• Independent • Likes to choose clothes with mom	'I like to get dressed myself every morning so that I look pretty'	'My mom helps me to get my clothes ready every evening'	Independent in dressing
Body temperature	• The temperature at home is normal, but likes to wear warm pajamas and blankets	'I feel cold at night sometimes'		Mild fever; some sweating
Skin and personal hygiene	• Doesn't like mom's help to have a bath, has a shower once/day independently	'My skin is often itchy after a bath, but not after a shower'		Dry skin Independent in hygiene
Avoid danger in environment	• Avoiding exposure to large crowds and people with infections		Routine cleaning of (contaminated) equipment/environment	Prevention of infections and re-infections
Communication	• Communicates with friends, via e-mail and phone when she has to stay home from school	'I miss my friends at school and in the neighborhood'	'I sometimes get sfrustrated with my sister and mom at home, because I don't see my friends'	Socially isolated
Religious matters	• No formal religious practice	'Sometimes I think:"how did God let this happen to me?"'		

Table 5.2/continued

ADL	Social systems	Perceptions	Interpersonal relations	Health state/assessment
Work/school	• Attends (normal) classes quite regularly; does not have special needs/assistance at school	'I feel sometimes that it is useless to go to school'	Occasionally loses touch with friends at school. Relationship with mom and sister strained through lack of outside stimulation	Watches TV/DVDs, uses internet/email a lot
Play	• Used to walk and play outside with friends or family members	'I like playing outside; fresh air helps, when I'm tired'		
Learning	• Good at school, motivated to learn new things with other kids	'I like reading and learning new things'	'I'm old enough to learn how to take care of my CF'	Motivated to maintain lifestyle

Table 5.3. Examples of the identified problems and goals	
Problem (i.e. reaction and interaction)	*Goal(s) (i.e. transaction)*
Cough at day/night times	Will be able to cough up mucus easily and privately
Decreased appetite/underweight	Will gain weight or remain the same
Feels socially isolated because of staying at home	Will be able to increase communication and social activities with family members and friends

(role). Anna thinks that she is a good big sister to Alice: they play quite a lot together, but she also appreciates the time with her mother, father, friends and classmates. Anna indicates that she has been using email more than before, because it has helped her to keep in touch with friends and classmates.

The information shared during the assessment is used to derive a nursing diagnosis, defined by King (1981) as a statement that recognises the distress, difficulties or worries identified by the client and for which help is sought. The nurse makes the nursing diagnosis as a result of mutual sharing with the client/ family during the assessment. The nursing diagnoses for Anna are shown the *Table 5.4*. These are derived from the interactions that occurred during the assessment. The care plan is composed of the problem(s), goal(s) nursing action(s)/intervention(s) and outcomes. The focus of the care plan is on the achievement of health through helping Anna to further develop interpersonal relationships with her social systems network, to take into account her own perceptions of her predicament and to maintain her physical health.

After the nursing diagnosis is made, the planning/implementation of interventions continues and outcomes/expected outcomes are identified. King (1997a, 2001) indicates that goal attainment is equal to outcomes. According to King (1997a) the concepts involved are decision making about the goals and agreeing to the means to attain the goals. She describes planning as setting goals and making decisions about how to achieve these goals. This is part of transaction and involves mutual exchange with the client/family. Implementation occurs in the activities that seek to meet the goals and it is a continuation of transaction in King's theory (1981). With Anna, the mutually established desired outcomes are shown in *Table 5.4*. During the discussion Anna, her mother and the nurse agree that Anna will be provided a quiet, single room for resting/sleeping and she will also be provided internet/email access in her room. Transaction would involve establishing and keeping a schedule of regular 'pulmonary toileting' and the nurse coordinating/

Table 5.4. Example of the care plan

Nursing diagnosis	Client goals	Interventions	(Expected) outcomes
Ineffective airway clearance	To slow down and prevent the decline of pulmonary functioning	• Respiratory assessment every 1 to 2 hours; pulse oximetry monitoring • Hydration assessment and fluid intake • Prophylactic pulmonary support: postural drainage: bed position; coughing assistance every 2 hours while awake • Teach: Coughing technique tissues and paper bag for disposal • Refer to respiratory therapist	The client will return to her level of pulmonary functioning prior to the onset of the mild flu; will successfully expel bronchial secretions with hygiene
Altered nutrition: less than body requirement	To ensure that the intake of calories meets the metabolic and physical growth needs	• A diet high in protein, fat, salt and calories • Nutritional (status) assessment: weight/height • Observe and document food intake (amount, type, calories) • Multi-vitamins; fat-soluble vitamins • Consult: dietitian to plan meals and nutritional supplement • Frequent, small preferred snacks available at bedside between the main meals (refrigerator in patient's room) • Mouth care prior to meals	The client will regain her appetite; her weight will remain the same or increase slightly
Altered family processes	To demonstrate greater awareness of stress and changing roles and relationships in the family	• Assess the effect of the patient's illness on the family • Help the patient coping and family identify strengths for coping • Provide information and teaching about CF • Encourage the patient and family to express their feelings without judging the expressed feelings • Encourage family members to participate in the patient's care • Initiate a care conference involving patient, family and members of the healthcare team • Facilitate coping and reaffirm patient's right to make decisions • Provide a referral to the CF support group	The client and family will gain an understanding of the client's condition and needs. The client and the family will start to identify personal and family strengths and regain a sense of control

providing referrals to the respiratory therapist(s), nutrition therapist and community resources for the family to identify appropriate support.

Evaluation involves descriptions of how the outcomes identified as goals are attained. In King's (1981) description, evaluation not only speaks to the attainment of the client's goals, but also effectiveness of the nursing care. She also indicates that the involved concept is goal attainment. The focus of interest regarding the evaluation is whether the goal was achieved or not, and if not, why not (King, 1997a). For Anna, the evaluation would include data/observations showing that her pulmonary function has returned back to the level prior to hospitalisation without re-infections/complications; that she has regained her appetite and maintained or gained weight; the family is well informed regarding the care of CF at home, and are confident and comfortable at discharge.

Applications and measures of King's Conceptual Framework in clinical practice

Hobdell (1995) reports a study that used King's interacting systems framework for research on parents of children with neural tube defect. The research investigated the relationship between chronic sorrow and accuracy of perception of a child's cognitive development as well as differences in that relationship for mothers and fathers. Sixty-eight mothers, 64 fathers and 69 children with neural tube defect participated. The study utilised King's framework and its findings have added essential information about prenatal response and the needs for usable information. The study showed that there was also a clear parental difference in both sorrow response and accuracy of perceptions. Chronic sorrow and inaccurate perceptions were demonstrated in mothers and fathers.

Ehrenberger et al. (2007) tested a theory of decision making derived from King's systems framework in women eligible for a cancer trial. The purpose of this study was to test an explanatory theory of decision making in women eligible for a cancer trial. The theory driven from King's framework proposed that the concept of uncertainty, role functioning, and social support related to emotional health (hope and mood state), which in turn relates to the treatment decision. A correlational study design was used to test the theory in a sample of 40 women. Findings provide empirical evidence of the adequacy of King's framework and supported, in part, theorised relationships among the critical factors. However, these factors did not illuminate the treatment decisions.

Reed (2007) reports a research study on social support and health of older adults. The aims of this study were to measure the reciprocal nature of social support from family and non-family members, compared to the amount of such support received, and to determine if social support was a predictor of health in older adults living in the community. The theoretical formulation was driven from King's (1981) Conceptual System related to the concepts of social support and health. It was hypothetised that social support would be a predictor of health for this population. The sample population included 140 older adults living either in their own homes or in housing for senior citizens. The instruments in this study measured perceptions of health, activities of daily living (ADL), instrumental activities of daily living (IADL) and social support. The primary hypothesis, that health would be predicted by the social support, was not confirmed. This may be because the older adults in the study rated their abilities to perform ADLs and IADLs very high. The findings of the study did not provide direct support for the credibility of King's Conceptual System most likely due to the limited number of variables in the model tested. However, the study and King's Conceptual System provide increasing knowledge about the health of older adults.

Newsom Wicks et al. (2007) report a further exploration of family health within the context of chronic obstructive pulmonary disease (COPD). This study focused on testing the theory of family health with a convenience sample of 140 patient caregiver dyads coping with COPD. Each instrument in this study was selected so that it was conceptually consistent with King's Conceptual System. The instruments measured the bronchitis emphysema symptoms, perceptions of burden, situational and family stressors, and family health. The findings of this study are important because they suggest that the proposed model has relevance for understanding general family functioning and family communication as dimensions of family health within the context of COPD. Family communication was impaired in this study sample. The results related to family communication as an indicator of family health reflect an extension of the findings from earlier studies.

Case studies

Husband (1988) has described how King's Theory of Goal Attainment can be applied to the care of the adult with diabetes mellitus. The author describes how the theory can be applied using the nursing process, which is the approach used by most nurses. They also note that the salient feature of King's theory is that it stresses patient participation in setting goals and planning care. For the diabetic patient population, this is especially important since, after discharge, they become their own health managers. Another interesting point that the authors underscore is the importance of diagnosing strengths and not just problems. If strengths and resources are identified, then the patient and nurse can build on these to overcome both current and future problems.

Alligood (1995) presents two clinical case studies that illustrate the utility of King's Theory of Goal Attainment in the nursing care of adult clients. She explains how the theory guides nursing practice using three dimensions of process. The first is the traditional process of assessment, diagnosis, planning, treatment and evaluation. The second dimension involves consideration of the concepts of the theory and provides content focus for the process of the first dimension. King's process of human interactions provides the third dimension with which the nurse assesses the level of communication occurring between the nurse and patient as nursing care progresses. The authors include both an acute and chronic orthopaedic case study and demonstrate the attainment of the goal and also the capacity of the theory to structure processes.

Daniel (2002) focuses on describing young adults' perceptions of living with chronic inflammatory bowel disease (IBD). King's Theory of Goal Attainment provided the theoretical framework for this qualitative, descriptive study. Through in-depth interviews, the participants had the opportunity to share their perceptions of what mattered most as they lived the experiences of this illness. The uniqueness and individuality of perceptions, the challenges of chronic bowel disease, recommendations for the future, and participants' expectations of healthcare professionals were explored. Persons with chronic IBD are faced with many life-disrupting challenges that profoundly affect their personal, interpersonal, and social systems. This research study supported the premise that understanding the patient's perspective and reaching perceptual accuracy through human-to-human interaction is critical to healthcare outcomes and achievement of the young adult's health goals.

Khowaja (2006) discusses the utilisation of King's interacting systems framework and Theory of Goal Attainment with a new multi-disciplinary model and clinical pathway. While not written as a case study, this article is nonetheless interesting to consider in this context. It is based on a study that was conducted in Pakistan and, as such, it speaks to the international applicability of King's work. The authors utilised it as a structure for investigating the development of a clinical pathway involving a multidisciplinary team. To that end, they applied King's Conceptual Framework, the Theory of Goal Attainment, and the transaction process model to the study. They found that King's work provided direction for nursing practice by emphasising the processes of multidisciplinary collaboration, communication, interaction, transaction and use of critical thinking. They concluded that nurses who interact with other systems can influence the health outcomes of the patients and families during their hospital stay and beyond discharge with the result that patients become their own health managers.

Empirical papers that have used King's framework

Froman (1995) conducted an empirical, quantitative study to explore the degree of perceptual congruency between nurses and clients related to the illness situation and the nursing care required. The specific concepts of perception and transaction from King's (1981) Theory of Goal Attainment were examined. The study was conducted on the medical and surgical units of three urban community-based hospitals. A convenience sample of 40 matched nurse–client pairs was used for the study. The data collection instruments measured patient satisfaction with care and the perceptual congruency. The findings of the study provided evidence to support perceptual congruency between clients and nurses as an important component of nursing interaction. In addition, the perceptual congruency appeared to be an indicator of client satisfaction with care. The findings provided support for the concepts of perception and transaction in the nurse–client encounter as outlined by King's Theory of Goal Attainment.

Rooke (1995) undertook a study to explore the concept of space in King's systems framework. This study was based on the critical incident method. Seven nurses described critical situations related to the concept of space. The situations come from their daily practice at a geriatric hospital. To reach saturation, according to the related situations, other experienced (medical, surgical, geriatric and intensive care) nurses and nursing educators were also asked to describe situations that could possibly be related to King's framework. The narratives addressed interpretation of different signs and reactions from patients regarding their experiences of space. It was obvious that the person's perception of space was related to the situation and the interaction between the actors. The study demonstrates how nurses can use the concept to describe and interpret their professional practice and how to achieve contextual understanding of King's (1981) definition of space. The narratives demonstrated also the importance of choosing appropriate strategies for space management and control, and thus provided specific implications for nursing practice.

May (2007) undertook a study to explore the relationships among basic empathy, self-awareness, and learning styles of pre-nursing students and to test the middle range theory derived from the nursing theory of empathy within King's Conceptual System. A total of 424 students participated the study. The instruments of the study measured empathy, emotional empathetic tendency, private and public self-consciousness and learning styles. The findings from the study provide initial support for the nursing theory of personal systems empathy, which was derived from King's Conceptual System. The findings suggested that basic empathy is related to self-awareness (private or self, and public, or body image) and all four measured learning styles (activist, reflector, theorist and pragmatist). The study revealed that diversity existed in basic empathy levels of the nursing students.

Suggested further reading

- Laben et al. (1991): This article illustrates how King's Theory of Goal Attainment may be used in conducting group psychotherapy with offender populations. The application of King's model is demonstrated in three milieus: an inpatient setting for juvenile sexual offenders, a state maximum security prison, and a halfway house for offenders involved in a work-release programme.
- Temple and Fawdry (1992): The problems faced by filial caregivers who are also health professionals have often been overlooked. A misunderstanding of roles and distortion in perception, for whatever reason, may influence the outcome of care. This article describes how King's theory provides nurses with a tangible and logical way of coping with the potentially debilitating effect of conflict between two roles or between two perceptions of a role.
- Norris and Hoyer (1993): In this article a neonatal intensive care unit provided a framework to test King's nursing theory. The framework of the study was based on selected concepts from King's Theory of Goal Attainment and literature on parenting. The article describes in an interesting way an attempt to move neonatal care from medicalisation of parenting toward transaction between parents and nurses.
- Hampton (1994): This article focuses on describing and discussing how King's Theory of Goal Attainment can serve as a nursing framework for managed care.
- Sowell and Lowenstein (1994): Quality care has long been described in the literature as an elusive concept. Healthcare services in community settings seem to demand new attention to the concept of quality. This article describes how King's Theory of Goal Attainment can provide a framework for the definition and delivery of quality care in community-based health services.
- Jones et al. (1995): In this article, the authors describe a discharge planning programme developed for geriatric and maternal-child nurses. King's Theory of Goal Attainment was used in the programme design. Evaluation methods include participants' pre- and post-surveys
- Murray and Baier (1996): In this article the authors describe how Imogene King's Theory of Goal Attainment was used as a theoretical framework for conceptualising the role and function of a transitional residential programme for severely and persistently mentally ill homeless individuals. The study utilised King's theory and associated

concepts of personal system, perception, communication, interaction, transaction, role, time, space, growth, and development.

- Tritsch (1998): The promulgation of managed care has become the catalyst for nursing leaders to develop creatively new approaches for the effective and efficient utilisation of resources. This article describes the application of King's Theory of Goal Attainment and the Carondelet St Mary's case management model in practice.
- Anderson and Mangino (2006): In this paper the authors describe how concerns about the traditional methods of communication between the various shifts were a catalyst for a nursing unit's decision to move to a more patient-involved model of shift-to-shift report. The article includes information on the benefits of bedside nurse shift-to-shift report, how one unit implemented bedside reporting, utilising King's Theory of Goal Attainment and some of the outcomes achieved after implementing this change at a 600-bed urban medical centre.
- Killeen and King (2007): The paper describes the development of middle range theory of the Patient Satisfaction with Nursing Care (PSNC). The author provides a very interesting examination of the concept and theory of PSNC for consistency with King's Conceptual System.

References

Ackermann M, Brink S, Clanton J, Jones C, Moody S, Perlich G, Price D, Prusinsky B (1989) Imogene King: Theory of Goal Attainment. In Marrinerr-Tomey (Ed) *Nursing Theorists and Their Work*. 345–60 St. Louis, Mosby

Alligood M. (1995) Theory of goal attainment: Application to adult orthopedic nursing. In M Frey, C Sieloff (Eds) *Advancing King's Systems Framework and Theory of Nursing* (pp 209–22). Sage Publications Inc. Thousand Oaks, California

American Nurses Credentialing Center (2008) *Overview of ANCC Magnet Recognition Program New Model*. Available at: http://nursecredentialing.org/Documents/Magnet/NewModelBrochure.aspx. Accessed: August 27, 2009

Anderson C, Mangino R (2006) Nurse Shift Report: Who Says You Can't Talk in Front of the Patient? *Nursing Administration Quarterly* 30(2): 112–22

Black J, Hawks Hokanson J, Keene A.(2001) *Medical-Surgical Nursing. Clinical Management for Positive Outcomes*. 6th edn. Saunders. Philadelphia, Pennsylvania

Carter K, Dufour L (1994) King's Theory: A Critique of the Critiques. *Nursing Science Quarterly* 7(3): 128–33

Daniel J (2002) Young Adults' Perceptions of Living With Chronic Inflammatory Bowel Disease. *Gastroenterology Nursing* 25(3): 83–94

Ehrenberger H, Alligood M, Thomas S, Wallace D, Licavoli (2007) Testing a Theory of Decision Making Derived From King's Systems Framework in Women Eligible for a Cancer Trial. *Middle Range Theory Development Using*

King's Conceptual System. 75–91

Fawcett J (1984) *Analysis and Evaluation of Conceptual Models in Nursing.* F.A. Davis Company, Philadelphia, USA

Fawcett J (2001). The nurse theorists: 21st century updates - Imogene M. King. *Nursing Science Quarterly* **14**(4): 311–5

Fewster-Thuente L, Velsor-Friedrich B (2008) Interdisciplinary Collaboration for Health Care Professionals. *Nursing Administration Quality* **32**: 40–8

Frey M, Rooke L, Sieloff C, Messemer P, Kameoka T (1995) King's Framework and Theory in Japan, Sweden, and the United States. *IMAGE – The Journal of Nursing Scholarship* **27**: 127–30

Frey M, Sieloff C (Eds) (1995) *Advancing King's Systems Framework and Theory of Nursing.* Thousand Oaks, CA: Sage

Frey M, Sieloff C, Norris D (2002) King's conceptual system and Theory of Goal Attainment: Past, present, and future. *Nursing Science Quarterly* **15**(2): 107–12

Froman D (1995) Perceptual Congruency Between Clients and Nurses. Testing King's Theory of Goal Attainment. *Advancing King's Systems Framework and Theory of Nursing* 223–38

Gulitz E, King I (1988) King's general systems model: application to curriculum development. *Nursing Science Quarterly* **1**(3): 128–32

Hampton D (1994) King's Theory of Goal Attainment as a Framework for Managed Care Implementation in a Hospital Setting. *Nursing Science Quarterly* **7**(4): 170–3

Hobdell E (1995) Using King's Interacting Systems Framework for Research on Parents of Children with Neural Tube Effect. *Advancing King's Systems Framework and Theory of Nursing* 126–36

Hockenberry M, Wilson D, Winkelstein M, Klein N (2003) *Wong's Nursing Care of Infants and Children.* 7th edn. Mosby, St. Louis, Missouri

Husband A (1988) Application of King's Theory of Nursing to the care of the adult with diabetes. *Journal of Advanced Nursing* **13**(4): 484–8

Husting P (1997) A Transcultural Critique Of Imogen King's Theory of Goal Attainment. *The Journal of Multicultural Nursing* **3**: 15–20

Jones S, Clark VB, Merker A, Palau D (1995) Changing behaviors. Nurse educators and clinical nurse specialists design a discharge planning program. *Journal on Nursing Staff Development* **11**(6): 291–5.

Kelsey Winker C (1995) A systems view of Health. In: M. Frey and C. Sieloff (Eds) *Advancing King's framework and theory of nursing.* SAGE Publications Thousand Oaks, California 35–40

Khowaja (2006) Utilization of King's Interacting Systems Framework and Theory of Goal Attainment with new multi-disciplinary model: clinical pathway. *Australian Journal of Advanced Nursing* **24**: 44–50

Killeen M, King IM (2007) Viewpoint: Use of King's conceptual system, nursing informatics, and nursing classification systems for global communication. *International Journal of Nursing Terminologies and Classifications* **18**(2): 51–7

King IM (1971) *Toward a Theory of Nursing: General Concepts of Human Behavior.* Wiley, New York

King IM (1981) *A Theory for Nursing: Systems, Concepts, Process.* Wiley, New York

King IM (1995a) The Theory of Goal Attainment. In M Frey, C Sieloff (Eds) *Advancing King's Systems Framework and Theory of Nursing* (pp 23–32). Sage Publications Inc., Thousand Oaks, California

King IM (1995b) A Systems Framework for Nursing. In M Frey, C. Sieloff (Eds) *Advancing King's Systems Framework and Theory of Nursing* (pp 14–22). Sage Publications Inc., Thousand Oaks, California

King IM (1997a) Reflections on the past and vision for the future. *Nursing Science Quarterly* **10**(1): 15–7

King IM (1997b) The Theory of Goal Attainment in practice. *Nursing Science Quarterly* **10**(4):180–5

King IM (2001) A nursing theory of personal systems empathy: Interpreting a conceptualization of empathy in King's interacting systems. *Nursing Science Quarterly* **14**(1): 80–1

King IM (2003) Assessment of Functional Abilities and Goal Attainment Scale: A Criterion Referenced Measure. In: O. Strickland and C. Dilorino (Eds) *Measurement of Nursing Outcomes.* 2nd edn. Volume 2: Client Outcomes and Quality of Care. Springler Publishing Company, New York 3–21

King IM (2006) A systems approach in nursing administration: structure, process and outcome. *Nursing Administration Quarterly* **30**(2): 100–4

Laben JK, Dodd D, Sneed L (1991) King's Theory of Goal Attainment applied in group therapy for inpatient juvenile sexual offenders, maximum security state offenders, and community parolees, using visual aids. *Issues in Mental Health Nursing* **12**(1): 51–64.

LeMone, Bruke K (2004) Medical Surgical Nursing. *Critical Thinking in Client Care.* 3rd edn. Prentice Hall, Pearson Custom Publishing, Upper Saddle River, New Jersey

May B (2007) Relationships Among Basic Empathy, Self-Awareness, and Learning Styles of Baccalaureate Pre-nursing Students Within King's Personal System. *Middel Range Theory Development Using King's Conceptual System* 164–77

Meleis A, Jones A (1983) Ethical crisis and cultural differences. *Western Journal of Medicine* **138**(6): 889–93

Meleis A (1991) *Theoretical Nursing: Development and Progress.* 2nd edn. Lippincott, Philadelphia

Messmer PR (2006) Professional Model of Care: Using King's Theory of Goal Attainment. *Nursing Science Quarterly* **19**(3): 227–9

Murray RL, Baier M (1996) King's conceptual framework applied to a transitional living program. *Perspectives in Psychiatric Care* **32**(1): 15–19

Newsom Wicks M, Rice M, Talley C (2007) Further Exploration of family health within the context of chronic obstructive pulmonary disease. *Range Theory Development Using King's Conceptual Syste*m 215–36

Reed J (2007) *Social Support and Health of Older Adults. Middle Range Theory*

Development Using King's Conceptual System. 92–104

Rooke L (1995) *The concept of space in King's Systems framework. Advancing King's systems framework and theory of nursing.* 79–96

Sieloff C, Frey M (Eds) (2007) *Middle Range Theory Development Using King's Conceptual System.* Springer Publishing Company, New York

Sieloff C. (2003) Measuring Nursing Power Within Organizations. *Journal of Nursing Scholarship* **35**(2): 183–7

Sowell RL, Lowenstein A (1994) King's theory as a framework for quality: linking theory to practice. *Nursingconnections* **7**(2): 19–31

Temple A, Fawdry K (1992) King's theory of goal attainment. Resolving filial caregiver role strain. *Journal of Gerontolgical Nursing* **18**(3): 11–5

Tritsch JM (1998) Application of King's Theory of Goal Attainment and the Carondelet St. Mary's Case Management Model. *Nursing Science Quarterly* **11**(2): 69–73

Walonick D (1993) *General Systems Theory.* Available at: http://www.survey-software-solutions.com/walonick/systems-theory.htm Accessed: August 27, 2009

Woods E (1992) King's theory on Practice With Elders. *Nursing Science Quarterly* **7**(2): 62–9

CHAPTER 6

Callista Roy's Adaptation Model

Introduction

Callista Roy began to develop her concept of adaptation as a framework for nursing while enrolled in the masters' degree programme for paediatric nursing at the University of California, Los Angeles in 1964. Her advisor, Dorothy E. Johnson, author of the Johnson Behavioral System Model, was very active in writing and speaking on the need to define the goal of nursing as a way of focusing the development of knowledge for practice. She encouraged Roy to build upon what she had observed and experienced with the resiliency of the paediatric patients who had been in her care. Her view of the person as an adaptive system grew from this early work and she first published an article on her emergent model in *Nursing Outlook* in 1970.

Also, in 1970, her model became the framework for a nursing-based integrated curriculum at Mount St. Mary's College in Los Angeles. Her collaboration with the faculty at the college provided Roy with important information that would help her to continue developing her model over time for both education and practice. With contributions from the faculty, Roy published three textbooks on the model (1976, 1984, 1991). In 1986, 1991 and 1999, Roy published collaboratively with Heather Andrews who added the valuable perspective of a nurse administrator to the advancement of the model. In 2009, Roy published her most recent book which not only built upon all previously published work on the Roy Adaptation Model but also included: a review, critique and synthesis of over 30 years of research based on the model; contemporary applications of the model reflecting current technology; and an explanation of Roy's philosophical and scientific assumptions for the 21st century with her newly added cultural assumptions.

In the preface of her 2009 book, Roy writes:

No other text on a nursing model has the vantage point of unifying and presenting model-based knowledge derived from more than 40 years of conceptual development and implementation in practice, education and research.

(Roy, 2009: v)

This is a notable point of distinction and the fact that the model has evolved over time differentiates it from many other conceptual models of nursing. In *Giving Voice to What We Know*, Picard and Jones (2005) share a dialogue that includes this from Roy:

> *I think the whole idea of convergence and the higher levels of unity are manifesting in many, many different ways... I think we were on the right track all the way along from Florence Nightingale, but it is just a terribly exciting time for knowledge. I think about the incredible science and philosophy of the 20th century, and then just taking that leap into the 21st century will give us all kinds of possibilities.*

Perhaps because her model is dynamic (i.e. it has evolved over time and responds to challenges in the current environment) and has a high degree of relevance to nurses practising in today's healthcare environment, it is very popular. In her 2002 book, *Nursing Theories*, Galbreath stated that 'few can fail to be excited by the explosive use of the Roy Adaptation Model in clinical practice, nursing administration, nursing education, and scholarly research'. In that text, the author listed 32 different types of publications from the early 1980s until 2000 that also includes papers reporting the use the model in countries such as Australia, Canada, Indonesia, Taiwan, Thailand, India, Pakistan and Sweden (Galbreath, 2002: 329, see also Tiedeman, 2005: 162–7).

The model's utility has been demonstrated in the literature in many different nursing situations and patient populations. Examples of some of the many writings on the application of the model are listed at the end of this chapter. Notable within this body of work are: Chao-Hsing's (2002) testing of the health-related quality of life theory, based on the Roy Adaptation Model, in Taiwanese children with cancer; Frederickson's (2002) use of the model for nursing knowledge development through research; Smith et al.'s (2002) discussion of the evolution of the caregiving effectiveness model to a midrange theory; Kiehl and White's (2003) study of maternal adaptation during childbearing in Norway, Sweden and the United States; Hsu's (2004) examination of concept mapping in problem-based learning; and Pejic's (2005) investigation of verbal abuse among paediatric nurses. Dixon's (1999) work is particularly interesting, since it makes the link between the model and community health nursing.

Roy herself described the model as 'primarily a systems model though it also contains interactionist levels of analysis' (Fawcett 1984: 248–50). She presents her four major concepts: humans as adaptive systems; the environment; health; and the goal of nursing, while also explicating the concepts related to each and their relationships. When reviewing and organising the publications that have featured Roy's model, an interesting observation was that there are several papers focused on: the concept analyses (Keil, 2004; Shin et al., 2008; Nicholson, 2009); testing the propositions and relationships between the concepts (Hamner, 1996; McVeigh, 2000); development of mid-range theories (Smith et al., 2002); and testing research instruments (Fowles and Horowitz, 2006; Ozkan and Ogce, 2009). These are also referenced at the end of this chapter.

Roy has based the development of her model on the scientific assumptions of von Bretalanffy's systems theory and Helson's adaptation-level theory. (Roy and Andrews, 1999; Roy, 2009). The philosophical assumptions are characterised by general principles of humanism, veritivity, and cosmic unity espousing a belief in holism and in the innate capabilities, purpose and worth of human beings (Roy, 1988: 26–34; see also Roy and Andrews, 1999: 56) (*Box 6.1*). It should be noted that Roy is a Catholic Sister in the order of Saint Joseph of Carondelet. It is possible to see in her work both assumptions and values that reflect her religious commitment and Christian perspective (see Roy, 2009: 30–2).

In 1997, Roy provided a redefinition of adaptation and a restatement of the assumptions that are foundational to the model (Roy, 1997). The most recent work, that has been called the Roy Adaptation Model for the 21st Century, takes into account transition time, transformation and spiritual vision. It is intriguing to see the development and expansion of the major concepts of the model over time and how this work has been influenced by the theorist's scientific and philosophical interests. The changes in philosophy that seem to have influenced her work include contemporary empiricism, postmodernism and increased relevance of the human need for meaning and purpose (Roy, 2009: 28–30). It is also notable that the development of the model and updating of the concept of adaptation has further led Roy (2009) to describe expanded philosophical and scientific assumptions in contemporary society and to add cultural assumptions (Roy, 2009: 27–320). The philosophical, scientific and cultural assumptions of the Roy Adaptation Model and their development are shown in *Box 6.1*.

The original Roy Adaptation Model was criticised by Fawcett regarding: the overlap and difficulty of distinguishing the adaptive modes (i.e. the self-concept, role function and interdependence modes); difficulty of distinguishing the external and internal environment; and the lack of distinct definitions for such key concepts as health, illness and wellness (Fawcett 1984: 264-78). As Roy developed the model, she successfully addressed this critique. However, the Roy Adaptation Model for the 21st century has expanded many of the concepts and made them far more complex than in the original model. The complexity of the concepts and terminology raises several questions: how well can inter-disciplinary healthcare team members

---

Box 6.1 Philosophical, scientific and cultural assumptions of the Roy adaptation model

Philosophical assumptions
- Persons have mutual relationships with the world and good/God-figure*
- Human meaning is rooted in an omega point convergence of the universe
- God is intimately revealed in the diversity of creation and is the common destiny of creation
- Persons use human creative abilities of awareness, enlightenment, and faith
- Persons are accountable for entering the process of deriving, sustaining, and transforming the universe

(Roy, 1997: 44; Roy and Andrews, 1999: 35; Roy, 2009: 31*)

Scientific assumptions
- Systems of matter and energy progress to higher levels of complex self-organisation
- Consciousness and meaning are constitutive of person and environment integration
- Awareness of self and environment is rooted in thinking and feeling
- Humans by their decision/human decisions* are accountable for the integration of creative processes
- Thinking and feeling mediate human action
- System relationships include acceptance, protection, and fostering interdependence
- Persons and the earth have common patterns and integral relations
- Persons and environment transformations are created in human consciousness
- Integration of human and environment meanings results in adaptation.

(Roy, 1997: 44; Roy and Andrews, 1999: 35; Roy, 2009: 31*)

Cultural assumptions
- Experience within a specific culture will influence how each element of the Roy adaptation model is expressed.
- Within a culture there may be a concept that is central to the culture and will influence some or all of the elements of the Roy adaptation model to a greater or lesser extent.
- Cultural expressions of the elements of the Roy adaptation model may lead to changes in practice activities such as nursing assessment.
- As Roy adaptation models elements evolve within a cultural perspective, implications for education and research may differ from experience in the original culture.

(Roy, 2009: 31)

understand these concepts; and does the complexity complicate rather than facilitate communication even among nurses? If it is desirable for a healthcare team to share an inter-disciplinary electronic health record that could include the patient, highly specific and specialised language could present a considerable barrier.

Nursing

Nursing is a knowledge-based profession which Roy defines as:

> *A healthcare profession that focuses on the life processes and patterns of people (and their interactions with the environment) with a commitment to promote health and full life-potential for individuals, families, groups and global society.*
>
> (Roy, 2009: 3; see also Roy and Andrews, 1999: 4)

Roy has pointed out that human potential may be limited by a lack of health and inadequate fulfilment of healthcare needs.

In her 2009 book, Roy revisits the origins of nursing with a discussion about Florence Nightingale. She notes that her aim was to promote health by using the environment to aid the natural processes of the body to heal itself. While she acknowledges that there have been many positive developments in healthcare that contribute to health and well-being, Roy also points out that there remain many unresolved concerns with healthcare delivery (Roy 2009: 5). As such, nurses need to know how to promote the health of their patients but also how to help them deal with episodes of illness in a changing and challenging environment. According to Roy, nurses can do this by promoting adaptation for individuals and groups to enhance environmental interactions. (Roy, 2009: 7; see also Roy and Andrews, 1999: 8–9).

Although Roy has continuously refined her definitions, there have been no major changes in the goal of the model except the explicit expansion of the theorist's perspective. In 1984, Roy (1984: 36–9) considered the goal of nursing in her earlier publication to simply 'promote adaptation'. According to Roy (2009:48–9), nursing's aim is to contribute to the overall goal of healthcare, which is to promote the health of individuals in society. It is then the nurse's role to promote adaptation in situations of health and illness and to enhance the interaction of the human systems with the environment, thereby promoting health. In keeping with the assumptions of the model, nurses aim to enhance system relationships through acceptance, protection, and fostering of interdependence and to promote personal and environmental transformation (Roy 2009: 48–9).

The nurse's role is to promote the adaptive responses in relation to the four adaptive modes (Roy 1984: 89–90). The modes, initially developed for human systems as individuals, have been expanded to encompass groups (Roy and Andrews, 1999: 48–51; Roy, 2009: 43–5). Today the modes are termed as: physiological–physical, self-concept–group identity, role function and interdependence (*Table 6.1*) (Roy, 2009: 89–103; Roy and Andrews, 1999: 48–51).

The adaptive modes

The physiological–physical mode for individuals and groups represents the category of behaviour pertaining to physical aspects of human systems. For the individual, the physiological mode has a total of nine components. There are five basic needs: oxygenation, nutrition, elimination, activity and rest, and protection. There are also four complex processes that are involved in the physiological adaptation. These are: fluid, electrolyte, and acid-base balance; neurological function; and endocrine function. At the group level, this mode pertains to the manner in which the collective human adaptive system manifests adaptation relative to basic operating resources (Roy, 2009: 48–51, Roy and Andrews, 1999: 43–5; see also Roy, 1984: 27–41).

The self-concept–group identity mode for individuals and groups represents a category of behaviour pertaining to the personal aspects of human systems. The basic needs identified for the individual are: psychic and spiritual integrity, the need to know who one is so that one can be or exist within a sense of unity. Self-concept is the composite of beliefs and feelings that a person holds at a given time. Components of the self-concept mode are: the physical self (including body sensation and body image) and personal self (comprised of self-conscience, self-ideal, and the moral-ethical-spiritual self). Identity integrity is the need underlying this group adaptive mode. The mode is comprised of interpersonal relationships, group self-image, social milieu and culture (Roy, 2009: 48–51, Roy and Andrews, 1999: 43–5; see also Roy, 1984: 27–41).

The role function mode for both the individual and group represents the category of behaviour to roles in human systems. This mode focuses from the individual's perspective on the roles that the individual occupies in society. The identified basic need underlying the role function mode is social integrity, the need to know who one is in relation to others in order to act. Roles within groups are the vehicle through which the goals of social systems are accomplished. The basic needs are: role clarity and the need to understand and commit to fulfil expected tasks so that the group can achieve common goals (Roy, 2009: 48–51, Roy and Andrews, 1999: 43–5; see also Roy, 1984: 27–41).

The independence mode represents the category of behaviour pertaining

Table 6.1. The four adaptive modes: physiological–physical, self-concept–group identity, role function and interdependence

Adaptive modes	Individual	Group
Physiological–physical	Needs: oxygenation, nutrition, elimination, activity and rest, protection Complex processes/senses: fluid, electrolyte, and acid-base balance; neurological function; endocrine function	Operating resources: participants, capacities, physical facilities, and fiscal resources
Self-concept–group identity	Need: psychic and spiritual integrity so that one can be or exist with a sense of unity, meaning, and purposefulness in the universe	Need: group identity integrity through shared relations, goals, values, and co-responsibility for goal achievement; implies honest, soundness, and completeness of identifications with the group
Role function	Need: social integrity; knowing who one is in relation to others so one can act; role set is the complex of positions individual holds; involves role development, instrumental and expressive behaviours, and role taking process	Need: role clarity, understanding and committing to fulfill expected tasks so group can achieve common goals; process of integrating roles in managing different roles and their expectations; complementary roles are regulated
Interdependence	Need: to achieve relational integrity using process of affectional adequacy, i.e., the giving and receiving of love, respect, and value through effective relations and communication	Need: to achieve relational integrity using processes of developmental and resource adequacy, i.e. learning and maturing in relationships and achieving needs for food, shelter, health, and security through independence with others

to independent relationships. For the individual, this mode focuses on the interactions related to giving and receiving of love, respect and value. The basic need in this mode is relational integrity, the feeling of security in nurturing relationships. For groups, this mode pertains to the social context in which the group operates. This involves private and public contacts within the group and outside the group. Two specific relationships are the focus within this mode for the individual: significant others and support systems.

For the group, the important components include context, infrastructure and resources (Roy, 2009: 48–51, Roy and Andrews, 1999: 43–5; see also Roy, 1984: 27–41).

According to the model (Roy, 2009; Roy and Andrews, 1999), adaptive responses are those that positively affect health, that is, support the integrity of the human [group] adaptive system. In the perspective of the model, human responses include not only problems, needs and deficits, but also capacities, assets, knowledge, skills, abilities and commitments (Roy and Andrews, 1999). All the responses are, according to the model, behaviour that can be observed. Nursing activities support adaptive responses and seek to reduce ineffective responses.

The nursing process

For Roy, the nursing process that aligns with the view of human beings as adaptive systems, assumes that the values and beliefs about people, environment, and culture are primary (Roy, 2009: 56). The nursing process is a vehicle or decision making method compatible with nursing practice utilising the model. Roy identified six steps in the nursing process:

1. Assessment of behaviour
2. Assessment of stimuli
3. Nursing diagnosis
4. Goal setting
5. Intervention
6. Evaluation

(Roy, 2009: 57–82; Roy and Andrews, 1999: 63–91;
see also Roy, 1984: 42–63)

Assessment of behaviour requires gathering data (in relation to each of the four adaptive modes) about the actions or reactions of the human adaptive system under specified circumstances and the current state of adaptation. (Roy, 2009: 58–62; Roy and Andrews, 1999: 66–71). Skilled assessment of behaviour and the knowledge to compare the person (or group) specific criteria are the starting point to evaluate behavioural responses as adaptive or ineffective. Ineffective behaviours are those that disrupt or do not contribute to the integrity of the human adaptive system in terms of the goals of survival, growth, reproduction, mastery, and individual and environment transformations (Roy, 2009: 59).

Assessment of stimuli (internal or external) requires the identification of that which provokes a response and places stress on the person's coping. Assessment of the stimuli uses the same skills as assessment of behaviour and this clarifies the nature of the stimuli. Stimuli may be: focal, meaning those most immediately confronting the system; contextual, meaning other stimuli present in the situation which may contribute to the effect of the focal stimuli; and residual, meaning any environmental factor within or outside the system with effects in the current situation which are unclear (Roy, 2009: 63; Roy and Andrews, 1999: 71–7).

The nursing diagnosis involves making statements that interpret the data that has been collected in the first two steps of the nursing process: the assessment of the behaviour and stimuli. Nursing diagnosis is defined as a judgement process resulting in a statement conveying the adaptation status of the individual or group (Roy 2009: 57; see also Roy and Andrews 1999: 66). Setting the diagnosis is the result of the process of critical thinking and judgement by the nurse. Roy (2009: 66) has suggested that the statement should identify and capture the behaviours with the most relevant influencing stimuli. The nursing diagnosis can also be a statement of adaptive responses that the nurse wishes to support. Roy (see, for example, Roy 2009: 69–76) has developed a typology of indicators for positive adaptation She has also indicated that the North American Diagnostic Association (NANDA) diagnostic categories may be related to adaptation problems and refers to these categories as clinical classifications (see, for example, Roy and Andrews, 1999: 78–81).

Goal setting is defined as the establishment of clear statements of the behavioural outcomes of nursing care (Roy, 2009: 76). Goals may be short-term or long-term relative to the situation. According to Roy (2009: 77) a goal statement designates not only the behaviour to be observed, but also the way the behaviour will change (as observed, measured, reported subjectively) and the timeframe in which the goal is to be attained. Roy (2009: 78) has emphasised that individual behavioural goals are aimed at the goals of adaptation that are in the model: survival, growth, reproduction, mastery and human and environmental transformations.

Nursing intervention(s) are planned with the purpose of promoting adaptation by focusing on both the stimuli and coping processes (Roy, 2009: 78; Roy and Andrews, 1999: 66). The nurse plans activities to alter the (selected) stimuli and uses strategies such as altering, increasing, decreasing, removing or maintaining. The nurse adjusts the stimuli by using the different strategies so that the stimuli fall within the person's ability to cope. The result is adaptive behaviour. Because many choices may be available to the nurse to alter the focal and contextual stimuli, Roy has suggested the use of a nursing judgement method developed by McDonald and Harms. First, relevant stimuli and coping processes are identified. Then, nursing intervention alternatives are considered in terms of anticipated consequences of changing each stimulus, the probability of the occurrence of the consequences (i.e. low, moderate, high) and the value of the change (i.e. desirable, undesirable). The use of this judgement method includes collaboration with the individual(s)/group of the human adaptive system (Roy and Andrews, 1999: 86–9; Roy, 2009: 78–81).

Evaluation aims to judge the effectiveness of the nursing interventions in relation to the behaviour of the individual or group. The nurse and the involved individual (group) look collaboratively at the behaviours to see if the goals have been achieved. Goal behaviours are compared to the client's output responses and movement towards or away from the goals are determined. If the goals have not been achieved, the nursing process begins again with questions regarding the accuracy and completeness of the collected data. The goals and interventions are re-adjusted based on the evaluation of the data (Roy, 2009: 81–2; Roy and Andrews, 1999: 89–91).

Health

Roy acknowledges that the concept of health is very complex. Her definition of health is integrally related to the human adaptive system and the environment as described in the model. She also notes that her understanding of health is deeply rooted in the scientific, philosophical and cultural assumptions that are the foundations of the model (Roy, 2009: 47–8; Roy and Andrews, 1999: 52–4).

Roy (2009: 48; Roy and Andrews, 1999: 53–4) has described human beings as adaptive systems, constantly growing and developing within a changing environment. From this perspective, health for human adaptive systems can be described as a reflection of this interaction or adaptation. In the model, adaptation has been viewed as a positive response of a human system that promotes survival, growth, reproduction, mastery, and person and environment transformation. Adaptive responses are seen to promote integrity or wholeness relative to the goals of the model, with the use of integrity to mean soundness or an unimpaired condition leading to wholeness. Health is thus viewed in the light of human goals and the purposefulness of human experience. In her latest book in 2009, Roy has defined health as… 'a state and a process of being and becoming integrated and whole'. This is a reflection of adaptation, that is, the interaction of the human adaptive system and the environment (Roy, 2009: 46–8; see also Roy and Andrews, 1999: 52–4).

Person

It is interesting to notice that the concept of person has evolved and expanded as the model has evolved. Although the theorist has always described the person in terms of systems and adaptation, the initial description and definition focused on the person as a bio-psycho-social being in constant interaction with a changing environment (Roy, 1976). Although Roy no longer uses this definition, the bio-psycho-social nature of a person as an adaptive system is still reflected in the four adaptive modes.

In the most recent literature, the person for Roy is a holistic adaptive system in which the whole is greater than the sum of its parts (Roy, 2009: 32; Roy and Andrews, 1999: 35–8). As a system, the person is a set of parts connected to function and the functioning requires the interdependence of its parts. Characteristics of the system include: inputs or adaptation-level stimuli; outputs or responses; controls or coping processes; and feedback. (Roy, 2009: 32–43; Roy and Andrews, 1999: 35–48).

Stimuli are defined as those that provoke a response and are further defined as focal, contextual or residual. Focal stimuli are those that are immediate, recognisable and draw attention in either a pleasant or unpleasant way. Contextual stimuli are those that contribute to the effect of the focal stimulus but are not noticed as the centre of attention. Residual stimuli are the environmental factors within or outside of the system that have an effect but may be unnoticed or even forgotten by the individual. Since the system is constantly interacting with the environment, the relevance of any one stimulus is subject to constant change (Roy 2009: 64-66; Roy and Andrews 1999: 38-40).

The human system responds to stimuli and this internal input is referred to as the adaptation level (Roy, 2009: 36–8; Roy and Andrews, 1999: 40–3). The adaptation level affects the person's ability to respond positively in any given situation. It is possible for the adaptation level to be integrated and well functioning, at which point the response system has been activated, or compromised whereby the system is weakened and damage has occurred (Roy, 2009: 36–8; Roy and Andrews, 1999: 40–3).

Behavioural responses to stimuli are the outputs of the human system. These can be observed, intuitively perceived by the nurse, measured and subjectively reported by the human system. Outputs of the system can be adaptive and help to promote the integrity of the system or they can be ineffective and threaten the system integrity. According to Roy, adaptive responses promote the integrity of the human system in terms of survival, growth, reproduction, mastery, and human and environment transformations while ineffective responses can immediately or gradually threaten the system. Ineffective responses can occur at the higher system level, such as in the family or in the group (Roy, 2009: 38–3).

Coping processes that are the system controls are described by Roy as innate or acquired ways of interacting with and influencing the changing environment. Innate coping processes are generally automatic and do not require thought or conscious planning by the person (Roy, 2009: 41–2;

Roy and Andrews, 1999: 45–6). An example is the body's temperature control processes, where perspiration is a response to heat. Acquired coping processes are learned through education or experience and are generally deliberate (Roy, 2009: 41–2; Roy and Andrews, 1999: 45–6). An example is the person's response to a drop in temperature as a stimulus which prompts the person to get a sweater and put it on and adjust the thermostat. Innate and acquired coping processes are also categorised into regulator and cognator subsystems. The regulator subsystem is comprised of basic adaptive processes such as chemical and endocrine coping processes. This responds automatically through neural, chemical and endocrine coping channels. Stimuli from the internal and external environment act as inputs and the information is channelled producing an automatic, unconscious response. At the same time, inputs to the regulator system also have a role in forming perceptions. A mother in labour provides an example of a regulator subsystem (Roy, 2009: 41–2; Roy and Andrews 1999: 46–7). The cognator subsystem is comprised of higher order cognitive and emotional coping processes. This system responds through four cognitive–emotional channels: perceptual and information processing; learning; judgement; and emotion. An example that illustrates all four cognitive–emotional channels is that of a person driving a car (Roy, 2009: 41–2; Roy and Andrews, 1999: 46–7).

Roy's model considers the regulator and cognator coping mechanisms to be subsystems of the person as an adaptive system, and innovator and stabiliser as control mechanisms inherent to the functioning of groups (Roy, 2009: 42–3; Roy and Andrews, 1999: 47–8). Stabiliser processes are those established structures, values and daily activities where the work of the group is done and the group contributes to the general well-being of society. The innovator sub-system is the second of the group control mechanisms; it identifies structures and processes that promote change and growth (Roy, 2009: 42–3; Roy and Andrews, 1999: 47–8).

Environment

For Roy, environment is the second major concept of her nursing model. She understands it as the world within and around humans as adaptive systems (2009: 46). Its current use within the model is that it encompasses all conditions, circumstances, and influences surrounding and affecting the development and behaviour of persons and groups with particular consideration of mutuality of person and earth resources, including focal, contextual and residual stimuli (2009: 29).

According to the Roy Adaptation model (Roy and Andrews, 1999: 51–2), human systems interact with the changing environment and make adaptive responses. Life is never the same for human beings. It is constantly changing, presenting new challenges and the human system has the ability to make new responses to these changing conditions. As the environment changes, humans have the continued opportunity to grow, develop, and transform.

When describing the concept of environment, Roy has drawn upon physiology/psychology and the work of Helson. Adaptation is described from this perspective as a function of the degree of change taking place and the human system's levels of adaptation. The three types of stimuli that make up the adaptation level have been described in the section 'person'.

Clinical application: Acute chest pain (angina pectoris)

Gordon Jones is a 58-year-old man. He has been married to Wilma for 30 years. They have no children. Both Mr Jones's parents have passed away and his father suffered a heart attack (myocardial infarction) when he was 55 years old. Mr Jones enjoys his busy, but stressful job as a sales manager for a local company, which occupies most of his time. Mr Jones used to smoke two packs of cigarettes each day but has cut down to approximately half a pack a day after several failed attempts to quit entirely. Mr Jones admits that he should not smoke, but it helps him relax during busy days. He has been moderately healthy throughout his life and he has only had mildly elevated blood pressure for the past three years for which he does not take regular medications.

One hot summer afternoon, Mr Jones was working on the back yard of their house, when he started to feel moderately strong chest pain. He decided to go inside the house, to sit in his favourite chair, and to 'relax' for a while. There was no radiating pain, but the left hand fingers felt numbed. The pain, not very heavy, continued for a couple of hours. During the afternoon, Mr Jones decided to go to the local hospital and get some help for the discomfort. On admission the doctor examined him and took an electrocardiogram (ECG). This looked normal (i.e. no ischaemic changes in the heart) and the physician gave him aspirin 150 mg, nitroglycerin spray and oxygen, and the pain subsided.

At the first level assessment, the nurse looked at the cardiac monitor that had been attached to Mr Jones. He had regular sinus rhythm; the p-QRS-t complex looked normal on the screen and his pulse was 80 beats per minute. His blood pressure was 160/70 mmHg. Mr Jones' skin looked pink/normal and he was obviously overweight. He expressed his concerned about the chest pain and worried that it could come back. Mr Jones' wife, Wilma, had been with her husband all the time and she was deeply concerned.

During the afternoon, when the chest pain started, a decrease of the oxygen supply to Mr Jones' heart muscle had stimulated pain receptors that transmitted the message of pain along sympathetic afferent nerve fibres to his central nervous system. The autonomic receptors of his lower brain then stimulated the sympathetic nerve fibres, and there was an increase in heart and respiratory rates. The result was an increase in the oxygen supply to the heart muscle. This increase can be viewed as a regulatory subsystem action.

Mr Jones had learned, from his father's experience, that left chest and arm pain could be related to his heart. His judgement was activated in deciding what action to take. He decided to go inside where there was air conditioning, to sit with his legs elevated, and to take slow, deep breaths. He decided not to call for emergency help, but he believed an adaptive response secondary to these actions would occur.

However, he may have been increasingly alert for further regulator sub-system output responses that might have caused him to question his decision. This represents the cognator process of selective attention and coding. Following the episode of pain, Mr Jones may have attempted to gain further insight into the causes of the episode. He may have decided that the hot weather was causal and remembered to limit his activities during extreme heat.

In this example, Mr Jones used the cognator sub-system processes of perception, learning and judgement. The stimulus that immediately confronted Mr Jones (focal stimulus) was the deficit of oxygen supply to his heart muscle. The contextual stimuli included the high temperature and physical work outside, the sensation of pain, Mr Jones's age and weight and the degree of coronary artery patency. The residual stimuli included his history of cigarette smoking and work-related stress and family history of cardiovascular disease.

For Mr Jones, the stimuli, adaptation level and coping process have resulted in an effective response at this point. However, the deficit of oxygen to his heart was a threat to his physiological integrity and maintaining his survival. This response became feedback to the system and a focal stimulus. Mr Jones used the cognator mechanism to adjust the total stimuli by going indoors to a cooler room and decreasing his oxygen needs by sitting down and elevating his legs. After the adjustment of the stimuli, the oxygen needs of his heart muscle were met, and the pain stopped.

At the first level and proceeding to the second level assessment, the nurse noticed that the chest pain had been relieved and that the vital signs were stable and within normal ranges. During the interview Mr Jones, his wife and the nurse started to identify areas of lifestyle/life that were important to explore. They discussed opening up areas of positive adaptation. It seemed necessary to consider factors such as his smoking, alcohol intake, diet and sedentary lifestyle (see *Table 6.2*).

The following problem (maladaptive behaviour) was identified: Mr Jones had life habits/style that were actually/potentially detrimental to his health, i.e. smoking, alcohol consumption, sedentary lifestyle, and weight.

Table 6.2. Assessments of the four adaptive modes	
Adaptive mode	*Assessment*
Physiological	• Had severe chest pain in previous 24 hours and numbing of fingers; no shortness of breath; no nausea
	• Weight: 105 kg, height: 165 cm
	• Pulse: 95/min, BP: 130/80 mmHg, Temp.: 36.7C
	• Smokes 10 cigarettes/day
	• Drinks in excess of 20–30 glasses of wine per week
Self-concept	• Slightly anxious, fearful of the return of the chest pain
Role functioning	• 58 years old; sudden change of role – sick role
Interdependence	• Active/not usually dependent on others

The nursing diagnosis for Mr Jones would be: increased risk for chest pain caused by a deficit of oxygen to the heart muscle associated with physical activities. The short-term goal(s) would read: Mr Jones will proceed with daily activities (behaviour) with no chest pain (change) after 30 minutes of rest (time frame). The long-term goals (adaptive behaviour) would be that Mr Jones will be able (1) to stop smoking cigarettes, (2) reduce alcohol consumption, (3) take part in a regular exercise programme that suits his capability and (4) reduce weight by five kilograms in six months (time frame).

Nursing interventions/actions: The nurse identified a need for information related to the heart disease and lifestyle (changes); a need for low-fat diet information; a need for cooking classes; as well as a need for a smoking cessation programme; and programme of cardiac rehabilitation exercise to increase cardiac strength and endurance. These plans of care alter the contextual stimuli and assist Mr Jones in reaching the long-term goals. The nurse judges the consequences of talking about a smoking cessation programme and cooking class to both Mr Jones and his wife Wilma as increasing the likelihood of starting/maintaining a low-fat diet and quitting smoking. The probability of success is considered high for the change in diet, since there is a class available at no cost at a community agency close to the Jones's home. In addition the value is seen as desirable to both Mr and Mrs Jones. However, the probability of success is considered moderate regarding the smoking cessation programme, since Mr Jones has attempted to quit several times before. The nurse, Mr and Mrs Jones select these intervention strategies along with others for implementation. The implementation requires that the nurse work with the patient and his wife, doctor, and the community agency. On the other hand, the nurse may find that the community does not have all the programmes. While exploring the alternatives with Mr

Jones, the nurse may also identify a community need to enhance the health of community members. The nurse then works with community agencies and groups, using the nursing judgement method to change this ineffective community response.

When Mr Jones was admitted to the hospital, he was experiencing strong chest pain and a life-changing event in his life. The chest pain was causing stress for a short while for all the four adaptive modes. Later on the nurse was able to consider the behaviours in the context of second level assessment identifying the areas that needed to be addressed. The identification of the problem(s)/nursing diagnosis was then devised from this assessment process. The short- and long-term goals were set to promote adaptation, that is, to increase Mr Jones' adaptive responses, to decrease ineffective responses and thus promote health. The areas of lifestyle changes were included in the care plan, but in Mr Jones' case it may or may not be possible to evaluate the achievement of these goals.

Testing and/or evaluation of Roy's model

Shyu et al. (2004) tested Roy's Adaptation Model by exploring the relationship between environmental stimuli, specifically barriers, and the mobility, and instrumental behaviours of hip-fractured elderly persons after surgery in Taiwan. A prospective study was conducted three months after hospital discharge with 87 elderly persons. After controlling for prefracture conditions, subjective environmental barriers significantly diminished the walking ability, self-care ability, and role performance of hip-fractured elderly persons. The findings of this study lead to suggestions for intervening with hip-fractured elderly persons after surgery.

Dunn (2004) describes the development of a middle-range theory of adaptation to chronic pain. The purpose of this paper is to present the strategies used to develop a middle-range nursing theory of adaptation to chronic pain based on Merton's description. Analysis and synthesis of the theoretical and research literature provided the foundational, theory-building strategies used to develop the adaptation to chronic pain model. Theoretical substruction was then used to deduce the adaptation to a chronic pain model from Roy's Adaptation Model.

Yeh (2003) conducted a study that examined the relationships among social support, parenting stress, coping style, and psychological distress in parents caring for children with cancer. The hypothesis that coping style plays a mediating role between social support and parenting stress, and psychological distress was tested for both mothers and fathers. In total, 246 mothers and 195 fathers of 270 children participated in the study. Structural equation modelling was used to test the hypothesis. The findings indicate that the hypotheses derived from the Roy Adaptation Model were supported for both mothers and fathers.

Tsai (2003) presents a middle-range theory of caregiver stress based on the Roy Adaptation Model as the first step in understanding the applicability of the Roy Adaptation Model in the context of stress in caregivers.

Smith et al. (2002) describe in their article the processes used to derive, validate, revise, and test the caregiving effectiveness model. Initially, the model structure and concepts reflect Roy's Adaptation Model (1991). Testing of this midrange theory used prospective longitudinal research with family members caring for patients requiring lifelong, complex, technology-based home care. The paper presents the conceptual critiques and statistical procedures, discusses derivation of model-generated nursing interventions and implications for use of these validation processes in developing nursing knowledge.

Chiou (2000) presents a meta-analysis of nine empirical studies based on Roy's Adaptation Model. The meta-analysis was conducted to determine the magnitudes of the inter-relationships of the four modes: physiological, self-concept, role function, and interdependence. Small to medium effect sizes between each two modes support the proposition of Roy's model that the four modes are inter-related. The only exception is the relationship between interdependence and physiological modes, as shown by the non-significant effect size. There are several limitations that should be considered when interpreting the findings of this meta-analysis. The study does provide a useful compilation of the Roy model's credible studies and proposes a direction for further research.

Case studies

Note: The Third Edition of *The Roy Adaptation Model* was published in 2009 and as of this writing case studies utilising this iteration of the model have not been published. However, the case studies referencing earlier editions may still be interesting and relevant to readers.

Gagliardi (2003) uses a case study to illustrate the adaptation of five women and three men diagnosed with multiple sclerosis (MS) by utilising the four model modes of adaptation (Roy and Andrews, 1999). The study focused on describing the experience of sexuality for individuals living with MS. This was a qualitative, naturalistic case study. The researchers interviewed the informants by telephone three times over the period of a year utilising a series of structured questions. The questions were based on the literature and the four modes of adaptation. The findings are consistent with the inter-related nature of the Roy Adaptation Model modes of adaptation (in particular, self-concept and interdependence) in that the themes overlap. As a qualitative, descriptive study, this is a very good example of the application of a research methodology consistent with the model.

Villareal (2003) describes a case study using Roy's Adaptation Model (Roy and Andrews, 1999) when caring for a group of young women contemplating quitting smoking. This article provides an overview of the use of the model by community health clinical nurses in Canada caring for a closed supportive group of three women who were in the precontemplation phase of smoking cessation. The model served as a guide to assess each member's level of adaptation in each of the four modes to identify actual or potential adaptation problems and then to examine the stimuli that influence those problems. Nursing interventions during six sessions focused on approaches to the management of stimuli to promote adaptation for the group by helping the members move to the phase of thinking of quitting smoking. The nursing interventions which aimed to help members change ineffective behaviours to adaptive behaviours enabled them to move from the precontemplation stage to contemplating smoking cessation. According to the author, exploring the group's thoughts and feelings about their nicotine dependency led to a more accurate understanding of their smoking addiction and of their perceptions of stimuli that produced the desire to continue smoking. It seems that the application of Roy's model is an effective guide for nursing practice when caring for nicotine-dependent clients.

Practice development papers based on Roy's model

Narsavage and Chen (2008) report a project that examined factors that predicted depressed mood at discharge and three months after discharge for 124 elders with chronic obstructive pulmonary disease (COPD). Roy's Adaptation Model (Roy and Andrews, 1991) provided the framework for the study. Three modes (physical, self-concept and interdependence modes) were identified and utilised for defining/operationalising the variables. The findings showed that the self-concept and interdependence mode variables of personal health competence, anxiety, daily functioning, and family emotional coping strongly predicted depressed mood for patients with COPD at discharge and three months later. Anxiety and personal health competence predicted depressed mood at discharge. In addition to anxiety and personal health competence, low daily functioning and ineffective family emotional coping were significant predictors of depressed mood three months after discharge. The authors link their conclusions and recommendations regarding the interventions back to the model. They propose that discharge referrals for home care services could be used to assess the four factors with the potential for the healthcare team to intervene. The recommendation regarding the interventions are that these could include anxiety reduction through music or other therapies, education to enhance perceived health competence, oxygen use with activities to improve functioning, and integration of informal caregiving support from the community to increase family emotional support.

McAllister (2005) reports a project that focused on promoting physiological–physical adaptation in chronic obstructive pulmonary disease (COPD), pharmaco-therapeutic evidence-based research and guidelines. Guidelines from the Global Initiative for Chronic Obstructive Lung Disease (GOLD) and evidence-based research include advanced pharmacological care for patients with COPD. Although clinical trials of medications have not supported evidence that long-term decline in pulmonary function can be prevented, pharmacological agents can reduce symptoms and prevent complications. High quality home care services may improve quality of life and prevent hospital admissions because of acute exacerbations. Roy's Adaptation Model (Roy and Andrews, 1999) was used as a framework in this project.

Frame (2003) reports a project that tested the clinical utility of the Frame Model of Preadolescent Empowerment as a means of enhancing the self-perception of children diagnosed with attention-deficit hyperactivity disorder (ADHD). The intervention, which has theoretical roots in Roy's Adaptation Model, Harter's Developmental Perspective, and Murrell-Armstrong's Empowerment Matrix, was administered to children with ADHD in a pre-test/post-test design in two groups (treatment and control groups). Findings indicate that this model significantly increased the perceptions of self-worth in pre-adolescents with ADHD. The findings of this study are limited due to a small total sample size of 65. The author concludes that the role of a school nurse, as facilitator of the group, is consistent with Roy's Adaptation Model.

Empirical papers that use Roy's model as the theoretical underpinning

Li and Shyu (2007) studied the coping processes of Taiwanese families during the post-discharge period of an elderly family member with hip fracture. The purposes of this study were to develop a conceptual framework explaining the coping processes of families after hospital discharge and to use the Roy Adaptation Model to examine the interdependence relationships. In-depth, face-to-face interviews were tape-recorded and transcribed verbatim. Data were analysed by grounded theory method. Findings revealed that a harmony between receiving and giving relationships was maintained by care receivers and caregivers during the post-discharge period to achieve an outcome of adaptation in their relationships. The researchers conclude that by understanding these coping processes, nurses can assist families to enhance adaptation.

Shin et al. (2006) report a study examining the relationship of maternal sensitivity to maternal identity, social support, maternal–fetal attachment and demographic variables. Maternal sensitivity is a mother's ability to perceive and interpret accurately her infant's signals and communications, and then respond appropriately. The conceptualisation of the study was guided by Roy's Adaptation Model. A cross-sectional, descriptive design was used. A convenience sample of 196 Korean mothers completed a self-report questionnaire. The findings showed that maternal–fetal attachment, self-identity as a mother, mother's employment status, identification with her baby, support from others, and infant's gestational age at birth were significant predictors of maternal sensitivity post-partum. It is concluded and recommended that providing social support, enhancing maternal identity, and facilitating maternal–fetal attachment in the antepartum period are crucial to improving post-partum maternal sensitivity.

Hunt Raleigh et al. (2006) studied family caregiver perception of hospice support. The purposes of this study were to explore hospice support of family caregivers in their decision to provide care at home and the relationships between hospice support, coping, and spiritual well-being. Roy's Adaptation Model was used as a framework in the project. Data were collected in home visits of 21 recently bereaved family caregivers of hospice patients using a set of questionnaires. Hospice workers were frequently identified as providing significant emotional support making the caregiver feel highly cared for, respected, and supported. Subjects scored moderately high on the spiritual well-being scale and reported low use of coping strategies. The findings of this study are limited due to a total of 21 respondents. The authors' link the findings back to the conceptual framework and conclude that both the hospice support and the spiritual well-being are contextual stimuli that influence the individual's ability to cope with bereavement and adapt effectively. The positive reports of hospice support and spiritual well-being and low use of coping strategies seem to suggest support for the hypothesised relationship among the contextual stimuli, coping efficacy, and adaptive responses.

Yeh (2002) conducted a study, the purpose of which was to test the Roy (1991) Adaptation Model-based theory of health-related quality of life in Taiwanese children with cancer. The environmental stimuli included severity of illness, age, gender, communication with others, and understanding of the illness. The severity of the illness was considered as a latent variable construct, including the stage of illness, laboratory values, and number of hospitalisations. Biopsychosocial responses, that is health-related quality of life, was hypothesised as a latent variable that consisted of (1) physical function, (2) psychological function, (3) peer/school function, (4) treatment/ disease symptoms, and (5) cognition functions. In total, 102 children with cancer participated in the study. The findings showed that the construct of severity of illness demonstrated excellent fit with the stage of illness, laboratory values, and total number of hospitalisations. The health-related quality of life also demonstrated good construct validity with five domains. The researcher concludes that this study support the Roy Adaptation Model-based theory proposition that environmental stimuli influenced biopsychosocial responses.

Suggested further reading

- Decker (2000) describes the effects of inflammatory bowel disease on adolescents. The author reports that limited studies/literature have addressed this issue, but several key concepts seem to emerge that point to ways for successfully dealing with these adolescent adjustment problems. The author describes how Roy's Adaptation Model provides a foundation for identifying and selecting interventions in working with adolescents and chronic illness. This paper includes interesting literature and a hypothetical case study.

- McVeigh (2000) investigated the relationship between satisfaction with social support and functional status after childbirth. Data were collected using the Functional Status after Childbirth instrument that has been developed by Fawcett et al. (1988) and this derives the role function adaptive models of Roy's Adaptation Model. Two hundred new mothers participated this study in New South Wales, Australia. Although no significant correlation was found between satisfaction with social support and functional status after childbirth, satisfaction with support from one's partner decreased significantly during the 6-month survey period, as did satisfaction with support from others. The researcher concludes that providers need to assess the social support needs of their clients and that a postnatal support plan could be used by mothers to negotiate the long-term involvement of others in household tasks and selected aspects of infant care. The findings of this study are interesting and important for clinicians.

- Zhan (2000) reports a study based on constructs from Roy's Adaptation Model. The researcher examined (i.e. tested hypotheses) the relationship between cognitive adaptation processes and self-consistency in 130 hearing-impaired elders. Data were collected through survey questionnaires. Results of this study supported Roy's theoretical proposition of cognitive adaptation processes and their role in the maintenance of self-consistency. Three cognitive processes (clear focus and methods, knowing awareness, and self-perception) significantly contributed to the maintenance of self-consistency.

Understanding these cognitive processes helps nurses to promote effective adaptation in older persons.

- Cook et al. (2001) conducted a study to explore the incidence and impact of physician verbal abuse on perioperative nurses. Roy's Adaptation Model was used as the framework for this descriptive, exploratory study. A schemantic model of variables and the concepts was developed. Seventy-eight peri-operative nurses completed the Verbal Abuse Scale questionnaire and 71 nurses reported experiencing some type of verbal abuse from a physician during the past year. Results show, however, that nurses use adaptive coping behaviours and problem-focused skills to deal with the abuse. This is an interesting study, but the findings are limited due to the small sample size.
- Niska (2001) reports an ethnographic study using Roy's Adaptation Model. The study was conducted among 23 Mexican American families in Hidalgo County, Texas. The purpose was to characterise the family goals of survival, continuity, and growth from the parental perspective during early family formation. This is an interesting qualitative study, providing more information regarding the use of the model in different cultures.
- Jesse et al. (2002) report an investigation that examined prenatal risk assessment from a comprehensive perspective to identify biophysical, psychosocial, spiritual, and perceptual factors in pregnancy affecting infant birth weight. Face-to-face interviews were conducted using standard and reliable questionnaires with a convenience sample of 120 pregnant women. Findings emphasise the necessity for nurses and other providers to screen for presence and source of social support during routine prenatal assessments. The Roy Adaptation Model was used as a framework in the study.
- Tanyi and Werner (2003) conducted a study that examined levels of and relationships between adjustment, spiritual well-being, and self-perceived health in women with end-stage renal disease. The sample included 65 women receiving haemodialysis. The women were fairly well adjusted to their illness; they demonstrated fairly high levels of religious, existential, and overall spiritual well-being and their self-perceived health was good. The Roy Adaptation Model was used as a framework in the study. The findings are limited due to a small sample size.
- Patton (2004) has examined the use of Roy's Adaptation Model of nursing within acute psychiatric nursing. After examination the author concludes that there exists a research gap in relation to the use of Roy's model within acute psychiatric nursing. It is recognised that Roy's model is well developed and therefore it has the potential to positively affect practice and patient outcomes within acute psychiatric nursing.

However, it is also acknowledged that a greater level of research-based evidence is required in order to fully justify the use of the model.

- Tracey and DeYoung (2004) conducted a qualitative study examining the effects of relocating to an assisted living facility in a select sample of elderly individuals. Small group interviews with open-ended discussion allowed participants to express feelings about their transitional experience and recall situations in their adjustment process. The study revealed a beginning of an understanding of the experience of moving and how to facilitate adjustment. Roy's Adaptation Model was used as a framework in the project.

- Pejic (2005) conducted a study investigating the experience of verbal abuse among a voluntary sample of registered paediatric nurses working in six hospitals in Eastern Ontario over a six week period. Roy's Adaptation Model (1984) was used as the conceptual framework for this study to examine external, focal stimuli to which paediatric nurses are exposed. A questionnaire was used to collect the data. An increase in stress level and decreased job morale were among the most frequently perceived personal and professional reactions of verbal abuse. The increased stress was explained by using Roy's model. The findings of this study are limited due to a small sample size (a total of 35 nurses).

- DeSanto-Madeya (2006) describes a secondary analysis of the meaning of living with spinal cord injury for the family using Roy's Adaptation Model. Seven themes emerged from the phenomenological study data. The findings of this study revealed that the meaning of living with spinal cord injury reflects all four modes of adaptation.

- Good et al. (2006) conducted a project on postoperative hypothermia. The authors report that nursing has contributed to the literature on hypothermia with studies on shivering and treatment modalities; however, the direct physiological consequences of postoperative hypothermia have been reported mainly in the medical literature. Evidence indicated that forced-air warming was the most effective method for warming hypothermic patients. The Roy Adaptation Model was explained as a framework for nursing care of patients with hypothermia. This is an interesting paper and it provides clinicians with practice guidelines for unplanned peri-operative hypothermia.

- Saburi et al. (2006) studied perceived family reactions and quality of life of adults with epilepsy in Harare, Zimbabwe. According to the authors, perceived family reactions refer to behaviours that occur in response to epilepsy. Roy's Adaptation Model was used to conceptualise quality of life in the physiological, self-concept, interdependence, and role-function modes. Face-to-face interviews were conducted on a convenience sample of 66 adults, aged 18–45 years. A three-part structured interview schedule was used. The findings showed that quality of life was not adversely affected in the physiological, self-concept, and interdependence modes but was affected in the role-function mode. Adults with epilepsy were uncertain about their families' reactions, such as overprotection, but felt accepted and supported by their families. Fear, isolation of the individual, secrecy, and concealment were negative strategies used by families and individuals to manage epilepsy. Roy's Adaptation Model was used to identify family reactions as significant and positively associated to the quality of life of adults with epilepsy. This study is very interesting example of the use of the Roy's Adaptation Model and its findings provide valuable recommendations for clinicians. The authors conclude that in order to enhance the quality of life in adults with epilepsy, nurses need to encourage positive family reactions such as openness, acceptance, and support, while discouraging fear, isolation of the individual, secrecy, concealment, and overprotection.

- Stewart (2006) conducted a narrative literature review focusing on sexual dysfunction in patients on haemodialysis. Roy's Adaptation Model was used to identify sexual dysfunction and its effect on adaptive modes in patients on haemodialysis. The findings revealed minimal patient expression of sexual dysfunction to healthcare providers.

- Bitner et al. (2007) describe in this paper a team approach to the prevention of unplanned postoperative hypothermia. A team of clinical staff members and personnel from the performance improvement department of a hospital used a performance improvement model to incorporate use of pre-operative forced-air warming blankets that resulted in improved postoperative core temperatures. Roy's Adaptation Model (Roy and Andrews, 1999) was used as a framework in the project.

- Hamilton and Bowers (2007) explored the experience of adult genetic testing. Grounded theory was used to plan, guide, and analyse in-depth interviews with 29 participants. The theory of genetic vulnerability was developed. The authors acknowledge that Roy's model of adaptation was a valuable lens through which to test and adapt this theory.

- Perrett (2007) examines the role of qualitative research in the development of the Roy Adaptation Model. The author explored the findings from qualitative research using Roy's Adaptation Model from 1995 to 2005 and compared this with the findings and recommendations from a previous review over a 25-year period (1970–1995). Findings from both reviews support the assumptions of the model while generating new information and demonstrating the valuable place of qualitative research in promoting nursing science.

- Thomas (2007) sought in this study to gain understanding of the influence of self-concept on adherence to prescribed regimens in individuals with heart failure. Roy's self-concept mode theory was used to examine the relationships between components of self-concept to recommended health regimens. The study also examined the extent to which aspects of self-concept cognitive perception of health regimens predicted adherence to such regimens. A convenience sample of 97 adults was collected from two large heart failure clinics. Three instruments were used in the study. The study is a good example of the use of the Roy Adaptation Model and it also provides interesting information for clinicians. It concludes that nurses need to identify methods that support feelings of challenge to body sensation, body image, self-consistency, self-ideal, and moral-ethical-spiritual self and minimise threat to body sensation, self-ideal, body sensation, and self-consistency to enhance adherence to health regimens in individuals with heart failure.

- Evans (2008) examined the feasibility of family presence in the operating theatre during breast biopsy procedures performed with local anesthesia, by ascertaining peri-operative nurses' attitudes towards the concept. Roy's model (Roy and Andrews, 1999) was used as a framework in the study. The participants completed a survey tool adapted from the ENA (Emergency Nurses Association) Family Presence and Support Assessment tool. The findings suggested that although nurses believed that providing emotional support was part of their job in practice, not all felt comfortable providing this support. The results of the study indicate also that the feasibility of instituting this intervention (i.e. support) would be challenged by system barriers. The respondents of this study, a total of 338 nurses were drawn from one AORN (Association of Perioperative Registered Nurses) chapter and thus the generalisability of the findings is limited.

- von Krogh and Naden (2008). The purpose of the study was to present the Norwegian documentation KPO model (quality assurance, problem solving, and caring). The model's professional substance, a conceptual framework for nursing practice was developed by examining, re-organising, and completing existing frameworks. The model's substantial elements/concepts are mainly derived from human needs theories in nursing (Henderson and Orem) and Roy's Adaptation Model (Roy and Andrews, 1999). Consistent documentation is arranged for by incorporating NANDA-I Nursing Diagnoses, Nursing Intervention Classification, and Nursing Outcome Classification. The model is interesting, since it can provide clinicians with a framework for documentation in step with legal and organisational requirements and at the same time retain the ability to record all aspects of clinical nursing.

- Kuchinski et al. (2009) conducted a systematic literature review. The purpose of the review was to determine if patients receiving treatment for cancer experienced less treatment-related fatigue if they participated in a regular committed exercise regimen, compared to those who did not exercise regularly. The review focused on 19 English-language studies from the United States, Europe, and Australia, conducted between January 2000 and October 2006. The Priority Symptom Management (PRISM) system developed by the Oncology Nursing Society was used for levelling evidence and the Roy Adaptation Model was used as a framework for the review.
- Mayne and Bagaoisan (2009) studied social support during anaesthesia induction in an adult surgical population. This project assessed whether there is a need for support-person presence during anaesthesia induction at an academic hospital. Roy's Adaptation Model was used as a framework for the project. The results of this project did not exhibit a significant need for a support person to be present during anaesthesia induction. The findings of the study are limited due to a small (69 respondents) sample size.
- Moreno et al. (2009) write in this paper about the Roy Adaptation Model and how it has been adopted as the frame of reference for the nursing curriculum at the Universidad de La Sabana School of Nursing in Colombia. The article discusses, through an example, the application process of the Roy model, the reflection that has been developed to study its central concepts and scientific and philosophical principles. The authors explain also the process generated from the model's application in teaching and practice.
- O'Mallon (2009) concludes that published research reports suggest further research with vulnerable populations, families, and persons from different cultures. The purpose of this literature review was to explore the concept of grief in the context of family adaptation. The Roy Adaptation Model is explored as an appropriate framework to guide future nursing research with bereaved families.
- Rogers and Keller (2009) describe in their article the development of a theory-based intervention to promote successful adaptation to an active lifestyle based on Roy's Adaptation Model. The paper discusses the critical elements of the Adaptation Model (i.e. spirituality, physical movement and self-efficacy) applied to the development of programmes and interventions to guide practice in health promotion in older persons. This article offers clinicians several ways to use the theoretical model to guide the development of a physical activity intervention for older persons.

References

Bitner J, Leana Hilde L, Hall K, Duvendack T (2007) A team approach to the prevention of unplanned postoperative hypothermia. *Association of periOperative Registered Nurses Journal* **85**(5): 921–9

Chao-Hsing Y (2002) Health-related quality of life in pediatric patients with cancer. *Cancer Nursing* **25**(1): 74–80

Chiou CP (2000) A meta-analysis of the interrelationships between the modes in Roy's Adaptation Model. *Nursing Science Quarterly* **13**(3): 252–8

Cook JK, Green M, Topp R (2001) Exploring the impact of physician verbal abuse on perioperative nurses. *Association of periOperative Registered Nurses Journal* **74**: 317–31

Decker J (2000) The effects of inflammatory bowel disease on adolescents. *Gastroenterology Nursing* **23**(2): 63–6

DeSanto-Madeya S (2006) A secondary analysis of the meaning of living with spinal cord injury using Roy's Adaptation Model. *Nursing Science Quarterly* **19**(3): 240–6

Dixon E (1999) Community health nursing practice and the Roy Adaptation Model. Public Health Nursing **16**(4): 290–300

Dunn K (2004) Toward a middle-range theory of adaptation to chronic pain. *Nursing Science Quarterly* **17**(1): 78–84

Evans L (2008) Feasibility of family member presence in the OR during breast biopsy procedures. *Association of periOperative Registered Nurses Journal* **88**(4): 568–86

Fawcett J (1984) *Analysis and Evaluation of Conceptual Models of Nursing*. FA Davis Company. Philadelphia

Fawcett J, Tulman L, Myers S (1988) Development of the inventory of functional status after childbirth. *Journal of Nurse-Midwifery* 33(6): 252–60

Fowles E, Andrews Horowitz J (2006) Clinical assessment of mothering during infancy. *Journal of Obstetric, Gynecologic, & Neonatal Nursing* 35: 662–70

Frame K (2003) Empowering preadolescents with ADHD. Demons or delights. *Advances in Nursing Science* **26**(2): 131–9

Frederickson K (2002) Nursing knowledge development through research: Using the Roy Adaptation Model. *Nursing Science Quarterly* **13**(1); 12–16

Gagliardi BA (2003) The experience of sexuality for individuals living with multiple sclerosis. *Journal of Clinical Nursing* **12**: 571–8

Galbreath J (2002) Roy Adaptation Model – Sister Callista Roy. In JB George (Ed) *Nursing Theories: The Base for Professional Nursing Practice* (pp 295–338). Prentice Hall, Upper Saddle River, New Jersey:

Good K, Verble J, Secrest J, Norwood B (2006) Postoperative hypothermia – The chilling consequences. *AORN Journal* **83**(5): 1054–66

Hamilton R, Bowers B (2007) The Theory of Genetic Vulnerability: A Roy Model exemplar. *Nursing Science Quarterly* **20**(3): 254–64

Hamner J (1996) Preliminary testing of a proposition from the Roy Adaptation

Model. Image: *Journal of Nursing Scholarship* **28**(3): 215–20

Hsu L (2004) Developing concept maps for problem based learning scenario discussions. *Journal of Advanced Nursing* **48**(5): 510–18

Hunt Raleigh E, Robinson J, Marold K, Jamison MT (2006) Family caregiver perception of hospice support. *Journal of Hospice and Palliative Nursing* **8**(1): 25–33

Jesse DE, Wallace D, Seaver W (2002) A holistic approach to risk-screening in pregnancy with Appalachian women. *Journal of Holistic Nursing* **20**(2): 133–51

Keil R (2004) Coping and stress. *Journal of Advanced Nursing* **45**(6): 659–65

Kiehl E, White M (2003) Maternal adaptation during childbearing in Norway, Sweden and the United States. *Scandinavian Journal of Caring Sciences* **17**: 69–103

Kuchinski AM, Reading M, Ayhan A (2009) Treatment-related fatigue and exercise in patients with cancer: A systematic review. *MEDSURG Nursing* **18**(3): 174–80

Li HJ, Shyu YI (2007) Coping processes of Taiwanese families during the post-discharge period for an elderly family member with hip fracture. *Nursing Science Quarterly* **20**(3): 273–9

Mayne I, Bagaoisan C (2009) Social support during anesthesia induction in an adult surgical population. *AORN Journal* **89**(2): 307–320

McAllister M (2005) Promoting physiologic-physical adaptation in chronic obstructive pulmonary disease: Pharmacotherapeutic evidence-based research and guidelines. *Home Healthcare Nurse* **23**(8): 523–31

McDonald F.J, Harms M (1966) Theoretical model for an experimental curriculum. *Nursing Outlook* **14**(8): 48–51

McVeigh C (2000) Investigating the relationship between satisfaction with social support and functional status after childbirth. *American Journal of Maternal/ Child Nursing* **25**(1): 25–30

Moreno M, Duran M, Hernandez A (2009) Nursing care for adaptation. *Nursing Science Quarterly* **22**(1): 67–73

Narsavage G, Chen K (2008) Factors related to depressed mood in adults with chronic obstructive pulmonary disease after hospitalization. *Home Healthcare Nurse* **26**(8): 474–82

Nicholson N (2009) Social isolation in older adults: an evolutionary concept analysis. *Journal of Advanced Nursing* **65**(6), 1342–1352

Niska, K (2001) Mexican American family survival, continuity, and growth: The parental perspective. *Nursing Science Quarterly* **14**(4): 322–9

O'Mallon M (2009) Vulnerable populations: Exploring a family perspective of grief. *Journal of Hospice and Palliative Nursing* **11**(2): 91–8

Ozkan S, Ogce F (2009) Psychometric analysis of the Inventory of Functional Status_Cancer (IFS-CA) in Turkish Women. *Journal of Transcultural Nursing* **20**(2): 187–93

Patton D (2004) An analysis of Roy's Adaptation Model of Nursing as used within acute psychiatric nursing. *Journal of Psychiatric and Mental Health Nursing*

11(2): 221–8

Pejic AR (2005) Verbal abuse: A problem for pediatric nurses. *Pediatric Nursing* **3**(32): 271–9

Perrett S (2007) Review of Roy Adaptation Model-based qualitative research. *Nursing Science Quarterly* **20**(4): 349–56

Picard C, Jones D (2005) *Giving Voice to What We Know: Margaret Newman's Theory of Health as Expanding Consciousness in Nursing Practice, Research, and Education.* Jones and Bartlett Publishers, Sudbury, Massachusetts

Rogers C, Keller C (2009) Roy's Adaptation Model to promote physical activity among sedentary older adults. *Geriatric Nursing* **30**(2S): 21–6

Roy C (1970). Adaptation: A conceptual framework for nursing. *Nursing Outlook* **18**(3), 42–5

Roy C (1976) *Introduction to Nursing: An Adaptation Model*. Englewood Cliffs, New Jersey: Prentice Hall.

Roy C (1984) *Introduction to Nursing: An Adaptation Model*. Prentice-Hall, Englewood Cliffs, New Jersey

Roy C (1988) An explication of the philosophical assumptions of Roy Adaptation Model. *Nursing Science Quarterly* **1**: 26–34

Roy C (1997) Future of the Roy model: challenges to redefine adaptation. *Nursing Science Quarterly* **10**: 42–8

Roy C (2009) *The Roy Adaptation Model* 3rd Edn. Pearson, Upper Saddle River, New Jersey

Roy C, Andrews H (1991) *The Roy Adaptation Model. The Definitive Statement.* Appleton and Lange, Norwalk, Connecticut

Roy C, Andrews HA (1999) *The Roy Adaptation Model* 2nd Edn. Appleton and Lange, Stamford, Connecticut

Saburi GL, Mapanga KG, Mapanga MB (2006) Perceived family reactions and quality of life of adults with epilepsy. *Journal of Neuroscience Nursing* **38**(3):156

Shin H, Park Y-J, Ryu H, Seomun G-A (2008) Maternal sensitivity: A concept analysis. *Journal of Advanced Nursing* **64**(3): 304–14

Shin H, Park YJ, Kim MJ (2006) Predictors of maternal sensitivity during the early postpartum period. *Journal of Advanced Nursing* **55**(4): 425–34

Shyu YI, Liang J, Lu JF, Wu C-C (2004) Environmental barriers and mobility in Taiwan: Is the Roy Adaptation Model applicable? *Nursing Science Quarterly* **17**(2): 165–70

Smith C, Pace K, Kochinda C, Kleinbeck S, Koehler J, Popkess-Vawter S (2002) Caregiving effectiveness model evolution to a midrange theory of home care: A process for critique and replication. *Advances in Nursing Science* **25**(1): 50–64

Stewarti M (2006) Narrative literature review: Sexual dysfunction in the patient on hemodialysis. *Nephrology Nursing Journal* **33**(6): 631–64

Tanyi R, Werner J (2003) Adjustment, spirituality, and health in women on hemodialysis. *Clinical Nursing Research* **12**(3): 229–45

Thomas C (2007) The influence of self-concept on adherence to recommended health regimens in adults with heart railure. *Journal of Cardiovascular Nursing* **22**(5): 405–16

Tiedeman M (2005) Roy's Adaptation Model. In: Fitzpatrick J, Whall A (Eds). *Conceptual Models of Nursing. Analysis and Application.* 4th Edn. (pp: 142–76) Prentice Hall, New Jersey

Tracey J, DeYoung S (2004) Moving to an assisted living facility: Exploring the transitional experience of elderly individuals. *Journal of Gerontological Nursing* **30**(10):2 6–32

Tsai PF (2003) A middle-range theory of caregiver stress. *Nursing Science Quarterly* **16**(2): 137–45

Villareal E (2003) Using Roy's Adaptation Model when caring for a group of young women contemplating quitting smoking. *Public Health Nursing* **20**(5): 377–84

von Krogh G, Naden D (2008) A nursing-specific model of EPR documentation: Organizational and professional requirements. *Journal of Nursing Scholarship* **40**(1): 68–75

Yeh CH (2002) Health-related quality of life in pediatric patients with Ccancer: A structural equation approach with the Roy Adaptation Model. *Cancer Nursing* **25**(1): 74–80

Yeh CH (2003) Psychological distress: Testing hypotheses based on Roy's Adaptation Model. *Nursing Science Quarterly* **16**(3):2 55–63

Zhan L (2000) Cognitive adaptation and self-consistency in hearing-impaired older persons: Testing Roy's Adaptation Model. *Nursing Science Quarterly* **13**(2): 158–65

CHAPTER 7

Betty Neuman's Systems Model

Introduction

Betty Neuman originally developed the Neuman Systems Model in 1970 as a framework from which to teach nursing students. Neuman and her colleagues evaluated the effectiveness of the model for two years (Neuman and Young, 1972) and it proved positive to the students' learning. (Neuman, 2002a: 327). She subsequently published an article on the teaching model (Neuman and Young, 1972) and then a chapter in Riehl and Roy's book on nursing conceptual models in 1974 (Neuman, 197–4). Her Systems Model has been widely accepted in academia and is often used as a curriculum guide for holistic and wellness-focused nursing education (Lowry, 2001). It has also been used successfully in education for other disciplines (Toot and Schmoll, 1995).

The model has been broadly accepted in nursing practice (Amaya, 2001). The literature is full of examples, in which the model has guided practice within many different settings such as acute care, home care, extended care and public health; within specialties such as surgical, obstetric, psychiatric and paediatric nursing; and within client populations such as the elderly, the chronically ill, the homeless, caregivers, and families. In fact, it has proven its relevance and applicability across cultural settings as well with published studies from South Korea (McDowell et al, 2003), Malaysia (Shamsudin, 2002), and Sweden (Lindell and Olsson, 1991), among many others.

The model has not changed fundamentally from its origination, but it has matured during use. Many authors have written about the model's utility in different settings which has lent creative interpretations to its propositions and resulted in the creation of many tools. The Neuman Systems Model (Neuman 1982a, 1989; Neuman, 2002b and see http://neumansystemsmodel. org/) resources provide an extensive bibliography of work that has been guided by the model for education, administration, and nursing practice. Overall, the model has acquired the characteristics of full development, or has matured as it has been used. Although Neuman's intent may not have been to develop a framework for all of the concerns of nursing, in fact researchers (Fawcett and Giangrande, 2002) and administrators (Sanders and Kelley, 2002) have successfully utilised its framework. Because the model provides a comprehensive and flexible structure, it can be adapted for use in almost any venue.

Interestingly, Neuman's model has so far had value in the context of an evolving and complex healthcare environment. With changes being driven by ever-developing technologies, increasing regulations, economic stressors and consumer demands, nurses are facing new expectations, roles, functions and conditions like never before. With this model, nurses seem to have a specific and unified approach to the process of giving care. It can also be claimed that, with the model, nurses have the structure to work effectively and creatively to incorporate changes into practice. However, this may perpetuate the work of nurses in a silo apart from other disciplines. In future, with demands for all disciplines to work in concert with the patient, the structure may prove too restrictive to allow for open communication and collaboration.

The Neuman model is a systems model which, in general terms, refers to the science of systems as described by Bertalanffy's General Systems Theory (Neuman, 1989: 11). Systems theory is the study of the nature of complex systems and a framework by which to analyse elements that interact. Its contribution is pragmatic as it sets forth a structure that depicts parts and subparts, their properties, patterns and inter-relationships as they comprise a complete system, in this case, the client or client system. The perspective in a system is multidimensional and dynamic as it simultaneously considers the interactions of component parts and the whole.

The model strives to be multidimensional and dynamic as it considers the person as a complete functioning unit. However, the approach of examining the subsystem(s) within a system reflects a reductionist perspective rather than a holistic perspective. Component(s) or variables exist within the model and, while the whole is recognised to be greater than the sum of its parts, attention to the parts and their inter-relationships may distract from its implementation as a holistic model in practice. This is a valid criticism of the model expressed by critics (see e.g. Fawcett et al, 1982).

A basic premise of the model is that wellness of the client is related to the response of the client to actual or potential environmental stressors. This is influenced by both Selye's theory of stress and adaptation (Neuman, 1989: 22) and Lewin's field theory (Fawcett, 1989: 67). It is interesting to note the diversity of the scientific disciplines from which Neuman drew inspiration, which also includes Gestalt theory (Neuman, 1989: 22), deChardin's philosophy on the evolution of life (Neuman, 1989: 22) and Caplan's (Fawcett, 1989: 67) levels of prevention. While none of the seminal work was done in nursing, Neuman's theoretical foundations and assumptions are nonetheless consistent with the humanistic and holistic heritage of nursing.

The Neuman Systems Model emphasises holism and nursing care that offsets the depersonalisation of technological aspects of care (Neuman, 1989: 10, 14–15; 2002: 10, 13). (N.B. The model has been consistently criticised since it is not seen as truly holistic, but reductionistic in its approach. The process requires that all client variables, personal factors, stressors and their relationships be analysed, which in practice may alone be quite daunting and difficult to accomplish. Once achieved, though, there then remains the act of transcendence beyond the sum of the parts to a holistic view and understanding of the client. Undoubtedly, there are practitioners who have been able to realise this ideal. However, it may be that many busy practitioners look at the pieces and perhaps their inter-relationships without ever seeing the whole.)

The problem regarding holism in the model seems to have its origins in another, also commonly expressed, critique regarding the clear definitions of the concepts in the model (for example, Fawcett et al, 1982: 39–40; George, 2002: 358–69). Recent nursing literature has also demonstrated the challenges of defining the concept of holism and its philosophical connotations. (see for example, Ham-Ying, 1993). The model values interventions that eliminate stressors prior to the manifestation of symptoms in the client and emphasises preventive care and wellness maintenance. In this regard, it is very well aligned with social trends and the changing demands of the healthcare system. Nurses who practise with the Neuman model as a tool for assessment and intervention(s) have the opportunity to transform the lives of their clients beyond just their physical health (see, for example, Russell 2002: 61–73). They can be powerful catalysts for change in the client's belief systems and in care modalities.

The model itself is highly structured and provides a framework for purposeful interventions that help the client retain, attain or maintain optimal wellness levels. The process of delivering nursing care is specific as the nurse identifies actual and potential stressors which may be moving the client system towards entropy. The model helps to clarify the relationships of elements of nursing care and provides role definition at various levels of nursing practice (Neuman, 2002b). The Neuman Systems Model has been described as a unique, systems-based perspective that provides a unifying focus for approaching a wide range of nursing concerns. In the literature (see, for example, George, 2002; Walker, 2005) the model has been considered a comprehensive guide for nursing practice, research, education, and administration that is open to creative implementation. It has also been claimed that the model has the potential for unifying various health-related theories and clarifying the relationships of variables in nursing care and role definitions at various levels of nursing practice. The multidimensionality and wholistic systemic perspective of the Neuman Systems Model seems to be increasingly demonstrating relevance and reliability in a wide variety of clinical and educational settings throughout the world (Neuman, 2002b: 3–33).

In 1988, Neuman established the Neuman Systems Model Trustee Group which defines its purpose: 'to preserve, protect and prepetuate the integrity of the model for the future of nursing' (http://neumansystemsmodel.org/index.html). There is also a Neuman Systems Model Research Institute with the purpose of formulating and testing middle range theories derived from the model. 'Researchers are invited to work collaboratively in groups focused on populations, middle range theory concepts, Neuman Systems Model concepts or methodologies. Scholarly work is concentrated on integrated reviews of the Neuman Systems Model-based literature to identify gaps in knowledge, as well as original multisite research projects'(http://neumansystemsmodel.org/NSMdocs/research_institute.htm). There is a biennial international conference with the 12th event being held in 2009.

Nursing

What is nursing? For Neuman, the central concern of nursing is the whole person, which is referred to as the client system (Neuman, 1982a: 8, Neuman, 2002b: 15–18). The goal of nursing is to promote optimal client wellness or system stability by preventing stress. Nurses coordinate client healthcare within an interactive client system. The nurse and the client mutually formulate and plan care that not only addresses symptomology but also the client's context and relationship with the environment (Neuman 2002b: 30). Through purposeful interventions, nursing helps individuals, families, and groups to 'retain, attain, and maintain a maximum level of optimal system wellness' (Neuman, 1989, 1995, 2002b). The nurse is seen as an intervener whose goal is either to reduce the client's encounter within certain stressors or to mitigate the perceived effect through implementation of appropriate interventions within the three levels of prevention, i.e. primary, secondary, or tertiary prevention.

- Primary: A stressor has been identified as a risk or potential risk but a reaction has not yet occurred. The stressor has not yet broken through the client's normal line of defence and, at this level, intervention retains health. The nurse's goals and strategies focus on mitigating client risk factors through interventions such as client education.
- Secondary: A reaction to a stressor has occurred. The stressor has penetrated the client's normal line of defence and, at this level, intervention attains health. The nurse's goals and strategies focus on the

nature of the disease process and interventions that target maladaptive responses.

- Tertiary: The client system has regained stability as a result of a secondary intervention. At this level, intervention maintains health. The nurse's goals and strategies focus on strengthening rehabilitative resources and ensuring progression within the current wellness state. This completes the cycle and leads back to primary intervention.

The nurse may be able to intervene at the primary prevention level by helping clients to strengthen their ability to respond to the stressor. This would be accomplished through (health promoting) interventions that expand the flexible line of defence and thereby help clients to retain system stability and avoid a stressor reaction. Secondary prevention interventions are undertaken when a stressor reaction has already occurred and are aimed at treatment of symptoms. The outcomes of these interventions are strengthened lines of resistance that protect the basic client structure and help the client to attain system stability. Tertiary prevention interventions are appropriate to help the client who has had a stressor reaction and been able to reconstitute or regain some degree of system stability. These interventions maintain the current level of wellness and prevent regression from the wellness level. The nurse serves as an active participant by supporting the client's defences and thereby assisting the client to respond effectively to the stressors. Nursing actions assist the client in creating and shaping reality in a desired direction. As such, in keeping the system stable, the nurse creates linkages among the client, environment, health and nursing.

The nursing process within the Neuman model consists of three components: nursing diagnosis, goals and outcomes (Neuman 1982a: 19; Neuman, 2002b: 29–30). The first is diagnosis that identifies, assesses, classifies and evaluates the dynamic interactions among five aspects that comprise the client system: the physiological, psychological, socio-cultural, developmental and spiritual. A proper assessment includes knowledge of all factors influencing a client's perceptual field and the meaning of any identified stressor is validated by both the nurse and the client. The diagnosis yields a nursing diagnostic statement that identifies actual and potential variances from wellness and available resources; that identifies interventions that augment existing strengths and help the client reach the desired stability or wellness; and that is a synthesis of relevant data and theory. Next, the client and nurse formulate nursing goals and strategies that assist the client in avoiding or adjusting to the effects of stressors. Nursing actions are initiated to retain, attain and maintain optimal client wellness using the three levels of prevention as intervention. (NB. This is, of course, a nursing model. However, the focus on nursing diagnoses which may not have meaning to care providers in other disciplines can be seen as a significant limitation. As several authors have written, other practitioners can learn and apply the framework of the model in their own practice. Unless they do learn to use it and to discern meaning from the nursing diagnoses, the documentation can be incomprehensible and can functionally concretise profession-centred practice rather than encourage partnership and patient-centred practice.)

Health

Health is a continuum with wellness or system stability on one side and variance from wellness or illness on the other (Neuman, 1989, 1995, 2001). Health is equated with living energy. Neuman (1995: 12) defines health/wellness as:

The condition in which all parts and subparts (five variables) are in harmony with the whole of the client.

Change is implicit in the definition of health given that achievement and maintenance of client stability/balance (i.e. energy available to the system) is related to the client's reactions to constant changes in the environment. A client's health may be at various levels within a normal range at any given point in time. There is a natural fluctuation throughout the lifespan because of the client's basic structures and adjustments to stressors in the environment. There is constant energy flow between the client and the environment and existing client system energy levels are a function of the actual or possible effects of stressors. (It is interesting to note the model definition, for example, in the second edition of the book in 1989: 48–50, does not give a definition for energy.) Wellness or system stability is attained, maintained or retained when there is more energy generated than is needed. This is referred to as negentropy (Neuman 1989: 11, 49). Conversely, when more energy is required than is being generated, the result is illness or death and is referred to as entropy. The degree of client wellness is determined by the amount of energy required to retain, attain or maintain system stability (Neuman 1989, 1995, 2001). Optimal wellness exists when system needs are met; unmet needs reduce the wellness state. The normal line of defence in the model represents the client's usual wellness level and this is the baseline against which variances are measured by the nurse (Neuman 1989, 1995, 2001). A client's degree of wellness is determined by how effectively client system variables react to environmental stressors. Health, then, is related to the internal, external and created environmental forces inclusive of genetic factors, past experiences and current perceptions. The return to and maintenance of system stability following a reaction to stressors is referred to in the Neuman Systems Model as reconstitution.

If health is a continuum with wellness or negentropy opposite illness and death or entropy, there is a necessary inconsistency with nursing as a practice of preventive interventions. It does not seem that the principles and goals of palliative care, for example, fit within this model and so the application is dependent upon how one interprets the concepts. However, attempts to apply the Neuman Systems Model in palliative care have been reported (e.g. Echlin, 1982).

Person

The Neuman Systems Model is based on the philosophy (ontological assumption) that each human being is a whole person that is layered and multidimensional. This is represented by a series of concentric rings or circles (see for example: Neuman, 1982a: 27). Contained within the layers are the five aspects of human beings, namely: the physiological, psychological, socio-cultural, spiritual and developmental. Although each of the variables is always present, they may appear in varying degrees of development and within a wide range of interactive styles and potential. Interestingly, the spiritual aspect was added to the model in the second edition of the book (1989) for the purpose of being more congruent with a holistic perspective of humans. According to Neuman (2002), the spirit controls the mind and the mind controls the body. It is an innate component of the person whether it is recognised or not. Spiritual energy is seen as empowering and something which can be activated at any time.

The person is referred to in the model as the client or client system (Neuman, 1989, 1995, 2001). This is because the model has a wellness focus

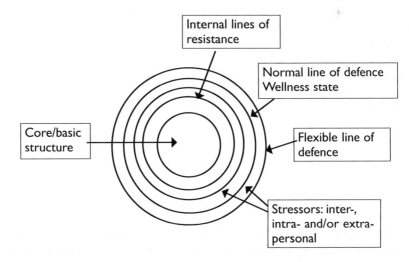

Figure 7.1. Graphic representation of the person/client system.

rather than an illness focus out of respect for the collaborative nature of the relationship between the client and the nurse. It is also useful to think in terms of a client system since the model can be applied to clients who may be individuals, a family, a group, a community or a social issue.

Each unique client system is a composite of factors and characteristics contained within a basic structure. This basic structure, or central core, is comprised of survival factors that are common to the species (Neuman, 2002: 17). These factors include such things as normal temperature, genetic structure, response pattern, organ strength or weakness, and ego structure. The core is surrounded by a series of concentric dimensions which protect the system from stressors. The flexible line of defence is the outermost boundary of the defined client system. It acts as a buffer to protect the normal line of defence, which is the usual wellness state. One's normal line of defence is dynamic, it evolves over time, and contains the client's normal range of responses to stressors and thereby reflects the client's usual wellness level (Neuman, 1989, 1995, 2001). This represents the client's ability to adjust to daily environmental stressors. Each client also has internal lines of resistance that function to protect the client's basic structure or system integrity. See *Figure 7.1*.

When lines of defence are penetrated or rendered ineffective to a stressor, the result is system instability which can manifest as illness. Closest to the core are the lines of resistance which are activated in response to a breach of system stability. When effective, the lines of resistance can restore the integrity and enable the system to reconstitute. If ineffective, the system moves toward entropy and perhaps death. The strength of the lines of defence and resistance depend upon the inter-relationships of the five aspects as well as on the nature and intensity of the stressor. (Neuman 2002: 17–18)

Environment

The interactions between the person and the environment and the continuous flow of energy between them are basic to the Neuman model. The environment is broadly defined as all of the factors or influences that surround the client system (Neuman, 1982a: 9, 18). Stressors are a prominent feature of the model. Stressors, defined as 'tension producing stimuli with the potential for causing disequilibrium' occur within the internal and external environment and Neuman (1989, 1995, 2001) has classified these as being intra, inter-, or extrapersonal in nature. Intrapersonal stressors occur within the boundary of the client system; interpersonal stressors occur between the client system boundary and one or more other client systems; and extra-personal stressors are those forces that occur outside of the client system boundary (Neuman, 1989, 1995; Neuman, 2002a). While stressors are inherently neutral or inert, they can have a positive or negative effect depending largely on the client's perceptions and ability to cope with the potential of a stimulus to cause system instability.

Both the environment and stressors are described within a similar typology. The environment in Neuman's model consists of the following typology: internal, external and created (Neuman, 1989, 1995, 2001). The internal environment is composed of those forces contained within the defined client boundary. All forces external to the defined client system make up the external environment (Neuman, 1989, 1995, 2001). The internal factors refer to intrapersonal factors that are resident within the client. In contrast, the external factors refer to factors that are outside of the client and may be either interpersonal or extrapersonal. When describing stressors, interpersonal refers to forces that are at a range close to the core, such as role expectations, while extrapersonal refers to forces that are at a range more distant from the core, such as financial concerns.

In 1989, Neuman added to the typology of the environment by naming an open system that exchanges energy with the internal and external environments and encompasses both. Like the addition of spirituality to the client variable, the concept of created environment is another example of Neuman's efforts to further delineate the holistic approach of the model. This created environment is inherently purposeful and is spontaneously formed by the client in order to maintain system integration, stability and integrity and to protect the client from inter-, intra- and extra-personal stressors (Neuman 1989, 1995; Neuman and Fawcett, 2001). It perpetually adjusts depending on the client system needs and represents the client's mobilisation of all system variables to ensure system function and wholeness. Neuman (1989) further describes the created environment as a 'process-based concept of perceptual adjustment' that functions to either increase or decrease the client's wellness state by unconsciously shielding the client from the true reality of a situation. It is possible to claim that this is a very important factor for the nurse to examine/assess carefully, since the created environment constantly changes energy from all system variables to maintain itself. The created environment, the nature and value of it, the protection it offers and the ideal that has yet to be achieved are all critical to consider.

At any given time, the client and the environment are simultaneously exchanging energy in the form of input, output and feedback. The interactions with the environment are circular and continuous even when a relatively stable state is maintained. The interactions of the client with the nurse then are to identify actual or potential stressors by type, time of encounter, and the nature and extent of the reaction. There can be any number of stressors at one time and the client's reaction to one impacts the reaction to all. The amount of resistance a client has determines whether or not a reaction occurs and to what extent. Adjustment of the system to a stressor may alter the client's response pattern and a stressor that was once harmful may no longer cause instability.

Clinical application of the Neuman Systems Model

The literature is rich regarding the applications of the Neuman Systems Model (Neuman, 1982b: 217–60; Neuman, 1989: 313–445; Neuman and Fawcett, 2002: 37–90). In the most recent, fourth edition of the Neuman Systems Model book, Amaya (2001: 43–60) has reported a systematic review of published papers that focus on the use of the model from 1974 to 2000 in clinical nursing practice. The review of this literature (107 publications) revealed that applications of the Neuman Systems Model to individual client care varied from simple comparison of the model concepts to complex detailed descriptions in a variety of specialty areas. A few publications addressed the application to family and community clients.

For our clinical case example, we have drawn a patient representative from our coronary care unit. The patient is a composite created to help protect and preserve the anonymity of individual patients while demonstrating the application of the model.

Case study

Client profile/biographic data: Mr Jones is a 66-year-old male who has presented to the admitting nurse with his wife. This is a re-admission four weeks after the client had coronary artery bypass graft surgery. At the time of the surgery the client was found to have elevated blood glucose levels that may precede the onset of type 2 diabetes.

Nursing assessment – identifying stressors: In order to obtain the necessary information about the stressors that are present, Neuman (1982b: 79) has suggested that six basic questions should be presented and answered by both the client and the nurse. In this way, variations in perceptions can be identified, discussed and reconciled. The questions were utilised in the nursing assessment for Mr Jones and the answers are presented in *Table 7.1*.

Neuman (1982b) includes problem identification and categorisation of the data as an important part of the assessment. In other words, the assessment focuses on identifying actual and/or potential stressors and their effects at intrapersonal, interpersonal and extrapersonal levels as well as the current strengths of the lines of defence. In Mr Jones' case an in-depth summary of the assessment is described in *Table 7.2*.

Nursing diagnosis. Neuman (1982a) emphasises that a clear statement of the problem(s) requires reconciliation of the perceptual differences between

Table 7.1. Assessment based upon Newman's Systems Model	
Patient's perception	**Nurse's perception**
What do you consider to be your major problem, difficulty or area of concern?	
The incisions from surgery several weeks ago are not healing very well. They feel painful to the touch and there is sometimes discharge	Feeling pain on both legs and chest at the incision sites; staples removed, no dressings; no signs of infection, wounds are healing slowly
How has this affected your usual pattern of living or life-style?	
It is painful to walk or even to stand on his leg. He had been active in his garden and had been accustomed to spending time with family, neighbours or with members of his church. Because he is feeling pain from both his leg and chest incisions, he hasn't felt like going out, participating in any activities or seeing any of his friends	Pain has restricted physical, social and personal activities Lethargic, irritable Anxiety from pain
Have you ever experienced a similar problem previously? If so, what was that problem and how did you handle it? Was it successful?	
He has not experienced anything like this in the past. When his doctor told him that his coronary artery disease had progressed to the point where he needed surgery, he took his suggestion immediately to have the bypass. He's surprised that he is having 'complications'.	Problem should have been identified earlier, during the hospital stay or at discharge to prevent current situation. No insight into recovery process at home
What do you anticipate for yourself in the future as a consequence of your present situation?	
He hopes that this can be resolved easily and quickly. He would very much like to get back to his active life and rejoin his friends and family as the happy and carefree man he used to be	Slightly unrealistic expectations of speed of recovery. No understanding of the required changes in lifestyle patterns or consequences of the elevated blood glucose levels and the risk of the onset of type 2 diabetes
Table 7.1 continues/	

Patient's perception	Nurse's perception
What are you doing and what can you do to help yourself?	
He has come back to the hospital. He feels that he has been doing what he was told to do relative to his recovery	Will need pain medication, physical therapy and education regarding diet (wife), exercise and lifestyle changes; unhappy about being re-admitted to hospital, but should be able to regain some aspects of self-care quickly as is well motivated
What do you expect caregivers, family, friends or others to do for you?	
He is relying on the caregiver's expertise to help him get beyond this 'complication'. His wife, family and friends are all very supportive. He doesn't ever want to be a burden or impose on others though. For the time being, he is also feeling affected by pain and worry and doesn't want to be short-tempered or irritable with anyone who is meaning to help him	Unrealistic hopes regarding problem solving and expectations that rely on healthcare providers. Good family support. Fear of losing independence and dislikes becoming a burden. Concerned about the psychological stress reactions that may impact human relations

the client and the nurse. In our example the two nursing diagnoses would be:

- Inability to obtain full recovery from surgery related to lack of knowledge and understanding of lifestyle changes including diet and exercise.
- Increasing social and spiritual isolation related to decreasing mobility and physical activities.

Goal setting and planning: The goal in the Neuman Systems Model is to keep the client system stable. The goal of stabilising the client system is achieved through the three modes of prevention (primary, secondary and tertiary). The planning is focused on strengthening the lines of defence and resistance. In our example, Mr Jones has experienced stressors that have penetrated the flexible lines of defence and are approaching the normal lines of defence. An outlay of the goals, interventions and outcomes for Mr Jones are shown in *Table 7.3*.

Evaluation. The nursing process is evaluated to determine whether equilibrium is restored and a steady state is maintained. Evaluation of Mr Jones' outcome goals following the interventions confirmed the outcome

Table 7.2: Summary of variables and sources of stressors	
Intrapersonal	
Physical	Slowly/non-healing wounds: AIC 11, blood glucose 21.0 mmol/l; poor diet and minimal exercise. Weight: 75 kg (weight gain after surgery: 2 kg). Height: 162 cm. TPR: 37°C. BP 120/70 mmHg, heart rate 69 (regular)
Psychological	He is worried about this 'complication' from the surgery but hopeful for a good outcome
Socio-cultural	He enjoys his family and friends. He likes to spend time with them being pleasant and carefree
Developmental	He does not seem to have realised that adjustments in his lifestyle are necessary to manage the elevated/high blood sugar levels that are factors in the wound healing
Spiritual	He is a devout and practising Christian
Interpersonal	
Physical	Since he left the hospital, his wife has been feeding him 'comfort foods' and his favourites without consideration for nutrition or special needs
Psychological	He trusted his physician and willingly went in for surgery. He is now feeling uncertain and fearful because the complications were completely unexpected
Socio-cultural	He does not want to be a burden to friends or family.
Developmental	Somewhat passive in approach to his health and prefers to hand over decisions and responsibility to caregivers
Spiritual	He is active in his church and has met with his pastor several times since his surgery
Extra-personal	
Physical	He has not been out and about as had been his habit
Psychological	He is becoming weary because of the duration of his recovery and is short-tempered
Socio-cultural	There are no financial barriers. He has supportive friends and family
Developmental	Lack of education/learning materials regarding the diet and exercise
Spiritual	He is not in contact with the congregation and community that are important to him

Table 7.3. Example of goal setting and planning

Primary prevention	Secondary prevention	Tertiary prevention
Goals Knowledge about diabetes and diet Weight maintenance Connection to his support system	*Goals* Lessen pain Regain mobility Increase wound healing Reconnect with support systems	*Goals* Increase mobility and return to usual activity level Follow a healthy diet
Intervention(s) Education for client and his wife Express empathy for the client relative to his worries and current limitations Encourage the client to maintain his relationships	*Intervention(s)* Assess severity of pain by using pain scale and provide pain medication Proper skin care Active and passive exercise and massage to improve circulation Coordinate with the pastor for prayer group to visit Motivate the client to be involved in his own care activities	*Intervention(s)* Physical therapy to exercise his leg and prevent recurrence of pain Refer him to the community diabetes resource centre for follow-up education and support Support the client and his wife towards the attainment of his goals
Outcome Demonstrate an understanding of the importance of diet Commit to a change to a low-glycaemic diet The client will feel relieved and more in control of his circumstance and healing	*Outcome* Pain free Good wound healing without infection or ulceration Able to interact with others normally without pain or worry interfering	*Outcome* His mobility and level of physical activity are back to normal He is eating well and is able to enjoy the company of others again He has a better understanding of his health concerns and how to keep them in balance

goals had been met and there was no need to reformulate for subsequent nursing goals. In the event that a client did not meet all of his or her goals, then new intermediate and long-range goals for subsequent nursing action would be formulated. Client outcomes validate the nursing process. NB. The emphasis on the client's perspective from the initial point of contact and assessment through to the evaluation of client outcomes is the strength of this model. It brings the perspectives of the nurse and client together in a collaborative effort towards the resolution of health-related issues.

Case studies

Campion Fuller and Hartley (2000) offer their perspective on the use of the Neuman Systems Model in the treatment of a young man with linear scleroderma (LS). While the disease is relatively rare, their case study provides an excellent demonstration of nursing care. Their nursing diagnosis identified stressors that included fear, self-concept disturbances and impaired mobility. Each of these stressors was addressed with interventions consistent with their nature.

Fear was related to a lack of knowledge about the disease and its medications. The nurses employed primary prevention and management techniques. This entailed active and open communication with the family, and education. The self-concept disturbances were related to the young man's feelings about body changes, social isolation and his physical appearance. The nurses employed secondary prevention and management techniques. They engaged family and friends to help the young man focus on what he could do rather than on what he could not do. They also helped to set him up with a home tutor and a support group, and encouraged positive emotions such as laughter, faith, hope and humour. The third nursing diagnosis was impaired physical mobility which was related to tight skin and contractures from the LS. The nurses employed tertiary prevention and management which consisted of negotiations with the young man about the requirements put forth by the physical and occupational therapists. After intensive rehabilitation, the young man was able to realise improvements so that he eventually had no new lesions and no further extension of old ones. Intensive inpatient rehabilitation does not really align with the definition of a tertiary prevention in the model. While it was a third step in the process, it was actually much more than simply maintaining reconstitution. As such, the author's ideas and interpretation of what constitutes primary, secondary and tertiary are an example of how application of the model in practice can drift from the original model.

Although not a typical case study, Melton et al (2001) present the process of completing a community needs assessment for a Sexual Assault Nurse Examiner (SANE) programme using the Neuman Systems Model. The authors used the model as the overarching conceptual framework for development of assessment guidelines that were also an adaptation of

Beddome's Community-as-Client Assessment Guide. The article offers the guidelines in a table format which gives clear and straightforward structure to analysis of the physiological, psychological, development, socio-cultural, and spiritual factors along with client perceptions. These are organised by intrapersonal, interpersonal and extrapersonal environmental factors. The project was ultimately successful but, perhaps equally importantly, the concise and ordered assessment guide reduced the amount of time, effort and money that was necessary to conduct the assessment. The authors point out that this presents an exciting opportunity for nurses to broaden their practice role and engage in health promotion and risk reduction for communities as well as individual clients. They go on to say that the process also supplies a unique community profile which can guide future direction for health planning, evaluation and research. This study was interesting and a good demonstration of the application of the model to a community.

Ume-Nwagbo et al (2006) illustrate that the client can be one person or more than one person. In their case studies, they look at both a newly wed couple experiencing marital stressors and an individual who requires coronary bypass surgery. They propose that nurses, who conduct their practice from a nursing theory base, while assisting individuals and families to meet their health needs, are more likely to provide comprehensive, individualised care that exemplifies best practice.

In the case of the newly married couple, the nurse's diagnosis was that a change in the couple's established patterns of living had led to unhealthy disagreements that penetrated both the flexible lines of defence and the normal lines of defence. This activated the lines of resistance which necessitated several preventions as interventions that included: a secondary prevention of marriage counselling to repair the normal lines of defence; tertiary prevention of re-education; and tertiary prevention of re-adaptation to establish new guidelines for their life together.

In the case of the individual needing bypass surgery, the nursing diagnosis, goals, interventions and evaluation were all multi-factorial. All of the variables were assessed and addressed but there was a focus on the interventions pertaining to the individual's physiological variable. There were many primary, secondary and tertiary interventions that effectively helped the individual to attain and then maintain optimal system stability. While the cases were very different, the authors illustrate how the basic holistic system was both comprehensive and flexible enough to guide nursing inquiry and care. While all aspects are considered in each case, this article illustrates that it is sometimes very appropriate to emphasise one or another over the others. In a model such as this, that considers multiple aspects simultaneously, there can be a difficulty in terms of prioritisation.

Kubsch et al (2008) illustrate the case of a woman suffering with interstitial cystitis. According to the authors, the literature states that there is no cure for the condition and that medical treatments can offer only symptom control. They had found a few studies, however, that had explored holistic treatment options. The authors suggest a protocol for holistic interventions that can be used to complement the medical plan and these include mind–body therapies that quiet the mind and help to relax the musculature of the bladder wall, energy therapies that unblock energy channels to the bladder, and spiritual interventions that provide a sense of hope and impart meaning to the sufferer.

While this case study reports only anecdotal evidence that holistic interventions can relieve the symptoms of interstitial cystitis, it is important nonetheless. Within the Neuman Systems Model, nurses are encouraged to apply their creativity to help clients attain, maintain and retain system stability. Relaxation therapy and meditation are examples of primary prevention interventions that can strengthen the client's flexible line of defence and prevent stressors from entering the system. Guided imagery, acupressure, and reflexology are examples of secondary interventions that can eliminate distressing symptoms. Journaling and the lived experience interview are some of the tertiary interventions that can help patients to maintain a state of wellness. This paper is interesting and important because it opens the door to non-traditional integrative modalities. While the article is well constructed and provides very good information carefully considered within the framework of the model, the big limitation is that the evidence is anecdotal. It would be very interesting to see a study examine this subject from a more rigorous and scientific perspective.

Suggested further reading

Comprehensive lists of studies, articles, etc. can be found in the Neuman Systems Model book that was published in 2002. The following suggested readings have been published since then and thus provide a list of the most recent papers on the use of the Neuman Systems Model.

- August-Brady (2000):This paper is an examination of anxiety research using Neuman's theory, prevention as intervention for clarity, simplicity, generality, accessibility and importance. The author finds that until such concepts as the flexible and normal lines of defence, the created environment, and the inter-relatedness of core system variables are further understood, the theory of prevention as intervention remains unclear.
- Torakis and Smigielski (2000): One of the greatest challenges in implementing the use of a nursing conceptual model is adjusting

current documentation to reflect the model appropriately. This article describes one organisation's process in adapting its documentation system to be supportive of the Neuman Systems Model.

- Norrish and Jooste (2001): This article aims at identifying crucial holistic aspects of nursing care of the alcohol-dependent patient.
- Shamsudin (2002): This paper discusses how a conceptual model developed in North America, that is, the Neuman Systems Model, can be adapted into the Malaysian nursing context. Because Malaysia is a multi-cultural country, adaptation, particularly of the concept of spirituality is important to consider.
- Gigliotti (2003): The credibility of the Neuman Systems Model can only be established through the generation and testing of the model-derived middle-range theories. However, due to the number and complexity of the model's concepts/concept inter-relations and the diversity of middle-range theories linked to these concepts, no explicit middle-range theories have yet been derived from the Neuman Systems Model. This paper describes the development of an organised programme for the systematic study of the model.
- Kottwitz and Bowling (2003): This article describes the development of the Elder Abuse Questionnaire (EAQ) to cover the five variables that Betty Neuman identifies as a wholistic system. The alpha inter-item correlation for the EAQ indicated moderate reliability for the new instrument to measure the perception of elder abuse.
- Reed (2003): This is an analysis of the grief concept using the Neuman model with perinatal grief presented as an example. The author believes the model is well suited to creating a guiding framework because concepts found in the model are similar to descriptions of the concept of grief.
- Skalski et al (2006): This integrative review using Cooper's five-stage method identified stressors in five patient populations. These data could form the basis for nursing practice as well as future research within a collaborative environment. Given the existing body of knowledge concerning Neuman Systems Model-derived middle-range theory concepts in the caregiver population, the middle-range theory of caregiver role strain could be tested empirically.
- Gigliotti (2007): This study's purpose was to improve both the external and internal validity of Gigliotti's model of maternal-student role stress in midlife women. These results support the propositions of the Neuman Systems Model as well as Meleis and others' transition framework.
- Moola et al (2008): This qualitative research approach (exploratory, descriptive and contextual) was used to explore and describe the stress

experienced by critical care nurses. The contextual framework adopted for this research was the Neuman Systems Model.

- Moscaritolo (2009): The purpose of this article is to provide clinical nursing faculty with the current literature related to humour, peer instructors and mentors, and mindfulness training as strategies to decrease undergraduate student nurse anxiety in the clinical setting. The Neuman Systems Model is used as a theoretical framework, and the application of this model to humour, peer instructors and mentors, and mindfulness training is examined.

References

Amaya MA (2001) The Neuman Systems Model and clinical practice: An integrative review, 1974–2000. In: Neuman B, Fawcett J eds. *The Neuman Systems Model*. 4th Edn. pp 43–60. Prentice Hall, New Jersey

August-Brady M (2000) Prevention as intervention. *Journal of Advanced Nursing* **31**(6):1304-1308

Campion Fuller C and Hartley B (2000) Linear Sclerodema: A Neuman Nursing Perspective. *Journal of Pediatric Nursing* **15**(3):168-174

Echlin D (1982) Palliative Care and the Neuman Model. In B Neuman (Ed) *The Neuman Systems Model. Application to Nursing Education and Practice*. pp 257–9. Appleton-Century Crofts/Norwalk. Connecutti

Fawcett J (1989) Analysis and evaluation of the Neuman Systems Model. In: B Neuman (ed) *The Neuman Systems Model*. (pp 65-92). 2nd edn. Appleton & Lange, Connecticut

Fawcett J (2002) *The Neuman Systems Model*. 4th edn. Upper Saddle River, NJ: Prentice Hall

Fawcett, J, and Giangrande, SK (2002) The Neuman Systems Model and Research: An Integrative review. In: Neuman B, Fawcett J eds. *The Neuman Systems Model*. 4th Edn. pp 120–49. Prentice Hall, New Jersey

Fawcett J, Carpentino l, Efinger J, Goldblum-Graff D, Groesbeck M, Lowry L, McCreary C, Wolf Z (1982) A framework for analysis and evaluation of conceptual models nursing with an analysis and evaluation of the Neuman Systems Model. In B Neuman ed. *The Neuman Systems Model. Application to Nursing Education and Practice*. pp 30–43. Appleton-Century Crofts/Norwalk, Connecutti

Fuller CC, Hartley B (2000) Linear scleroderma: A Neuman nursing perspective. *Journal of Pediatric Nursing* **15**(3): 168–74

George JB (2002) The Neuman Systems Model. In: J George ed. *Nursing Theories The Base for Professional Nursing Practice*. 5th edn. pp 339–84. Prentice Hall, New Jersey

Gigliotti E (2003) The Neuman Systems Model Institute: Testing middle-range theories. *Nursing Science Quarterly* **16**(3): 201–6

Gigliotti E (2007) Improving external and internal validity of a model of midlife women's maternal-student role stress. *Nursing Science Quarterly* **20**(2): 161–

70

Ham-Ying S (1993) Analysis of the concept of holism within the context of nursing. *British Journal of Nursing* **2**(15): 771–5

Kottwitz D, Bowling S (2003) A pilot study of the elder abuse questionnaire. *Kansas Nurse* **78**(7): 4–6

Kubsch S, Linton S, Hankerson C, Wichowski H (2008)Holistic Interventions Protocol for Interstitial Cystitis Symptoms Control. *Holistic Nursing Practice*. **July/August**: 183–90

Lindell M, Olsson H (1991) Can combined oral contraceptives be made more effective by means of a nursing care model? *Journal Advanced Nursing* **16**(4): 475–9

Lowry L (2001) The Neuman Systems Model and Education: An Integrative Review. In: Neuman B, Fawcett J eds. *The Neuman Systems Model*. 4th Edn. pp 216–37. Prentice Hall, New Jersey

McDowell BM, Chang NJ, Choi SS (2003) Children's health retention in South Korea and the United Stated: A cross-cultural comparison. *Journal of Pediatric Nursing* **18**(6): 409–15

Melton L, Secrest J, Chien A, Andersen B (2001) A community needs assessment for a SANE Program using Neuman's Model. *Journal of the American Academy of Nurse Practitioners* **13**(4): 178–86

Moola S, Ehlers VJ, Hattingh SP (2008) Critical care nurses' perceptions of stress and stress-related situations in the workplace. *Curationis* **31**(2): 77–86

Moscaritolo LM (2009) Interventional strategies to decrease nursing student anxiety in the clinical learning environment. *Journal of Nursing Education* **48**(1): 17–23

Neuman B (1974) The Betty Neuman health-care Systems Model: A total person approach to client problems. In JP Riehl, C Roy eds. *Conceptual Models for Nursing Practice*. pp 94–104. Appleton-Century-Crofts, New York

Neuman B (1982a) The Systems concept and nursing. In B Neuman ed. *The Neuman Systems Model. Application to Nursing Education and Practice*. pp 3–7. Appleton-Century Crofts, Norwalk, Connecutti

Neuman B (1982b) The Neuman health-care Systems Model: A total approach to client care. In B Neuman ed. *The Neuman Systems Model. Application to Nursing Education and Practice*. pp 8–29. Appleton-Century Crofts, Norwalk, Connecutti

Neuman BM (1989) The Neuman Systems Model. In B Nuuman ed. *The Neuman Systems Model*. (pp 3–50.) 2nd Edn. Appleton and Lange, Norwalk, CT

Neuman B (1995) *The Neuman Systems Model*. 3rd edn. Appleton & Lange, Norwalk

Neuman B (2002a) Betty Neuman's autobiography and chronology of the development and utilization of the Neuman Systems Model. In B Neuman, J Fawcett (eds) *The Neuman Systems Model* (pp 325–46). 4th edn. Prentice Hall, New Jersey

Neuman B. (2002b) The Neuman Systems Model. In: B Neuman, J Fawcett (eds) *The Neuman Systems Model* (pp 3–33). 4th edn. Prentice Hall, New Jersey

Neuman B, Young, RJ (1972) A model for teaching total person approach to client problems. *Nursing Research* **21**: 264–9

Norrish ME, Jooste K (2001) Nursing care of the patient undergoing alcohol detoxification. *Curationis* **24**(3): 36–48

Reed K (2003) Grief is more than tears. *Nursing Science Quarterly* **16**(1): 77–81

Russell J (2002) The Neuman Systems Model and Clinical Tools. In Neuman B, Fawcett J eds. *The Neuman Systems Model*. 4th edn. pp 61–73. Prentice Hall New Jersey

Sanders NF, Kelley JA (2002) The Neuman Systems Model and Administration of Nursing Services. An Integrative review In Neuman B, Fawcett J eds. *The Neuman Systems Model*. 4th Edn. pp 271–87. Prentice Hall, New Jersey

Shamsudin N (2002) Can the Neuman Systems Model be adapted to the Malasyian nursing context? *International Journal of Nursing Practice* **8**(2): 99–105

Skalski CA, DiGerolamo L, Gigliotti E (2006) Stressors in five client populations: Neuman Systems Model-based literature review. *Journal of Advanced Nursing* **56**(1): 69–78

Toot JL, Schmoll BJ (1995) The Neuman Systems Model and physical therapy education curricula. In B Neuman ed. *The Neuman Systems Model*. pp 231–46. Appleton and Lange, Norwalk, CT

Torakis ML, Smigielski CM (2000) Documentation of model-based practice: One hospital's experience. *Pediatric Nurse* **26**(4): 394–7

Ume-Nwagbo P, DeWan S, Lowry L (2006) Using the Neuman Systems Model for best practices. *Nursing Science Quarterly* **19**(1): 31–5

Walker P (2005) Neuman's System Model. In J Fitzpatrick, A Whall eds. *Conceptual Models of Nursing. Analaysis and Application*. Pearson Prentice Hall, New Jersey.

CHAPTER 8

Dorothea Orem's Self-Care Model

One nursing model that is widely used in North America (deMontigny et al, 1997; Timmins and Horan, 2001) and in other parts of the world (see McKenna and Slevin, 2007) is Dorothea Orem's Self-Care Model. Orem declares in her own words that her model is a comprehensive theory of nursing (and a conceptual framework); one that was first expressed by the author in 1958 and subsequently captured in the first publication of her book *Nursing: Concepts of Practice* in 1971. Having undergone several revisions and developments, the fifth edition of this book was published in 1995. The model has been adopted as an underpinning philosophy for some nursing programme curricula (Timmins and Horan, 2001), has a well-established utility for guiding certain aspects of clinical practice (Aish and Isenberg, 1996; Gaffney and Moore, 1996, Soderhamn and Cliffordson, 2001; Allison, 2007) and is frequently used as the theoretical framework upon which nursing-focused research studies are based (see for example, Geden and Taylor, 1999; Campbell and Weber, 2000; Dalton et al, 2006). Given the widespread successful application of this model and the body of empirical evidence which highlights how the model can guide flourishing practice development initiatives, the authors would assert that Orem's work should be considered as one of the most influential examples of grand level nursing theories.

Orem (1980) argues that a crucial and yet fundamental question facing all nurses, is when and why people can be helped through nursing, as distinguished from other forms of human service. In answering this question, Orem (1980) says, nurses will be able to identify the proper focus of their practice; it indicates the boundaries of nursing practice (which implies that some nurses may have been engaged in practice that was, for Orem at least, an improper focus for nurses), and identifies the object of nursing knowledge and thus those with whom legitimate and proper therapeutic relationship can/should be established. (While the authors wholeheartedly concur with Orem's view regarding the need to establish the boundaries for the 'proper' focus of nursing, we would add a caveat that these boundaries are not fixed indelibly; they change over time and vary across different cultures and countries.) For Orem (1980: 27), a central premise of nursing is that:

> *People can benefit from nursing because they are subject to health-related*
> *or health-derived limitations that render them incapable of continuous*
> *self-care or dependent care.*

For Orem, social groups throughout history have provided nursing to those in need of such contact and communication. She declares that this is the first prerequisite for nursing to occur, the others being a willingness on behalf of both those who need nursing, and those who offer i t, to enter into and maintain legitimate interpersonal relationships, and an understanding gained through this relationship, of how and to what extent the patient might be helped through the action of nursing.

Orem (1980: 3) asserts that nursing occurs in four categories: (1) home nursing (where the nurse enters the home of the patient), (2) adult ambulatory nursing (where the patient visits the nurse and returns home following the visit), (3) infant/child nursing (where the parent/guardian brings the child to the nurse and returns home following the visit and, (4) hospital/long-term, extended care nursing (where nurses come to a healthcare institution where patients of any age are in residence). While this may seem a little quaint to the nurse of the 21st century who encounters and/or engages in nursing in a much wider range of settings (Royal College of Nursing, 2009), Orem's grasp of the growing number of settings/contexts in which nursing was occurring in the 1970s suggests she had an awareness of the (ever) changing scope of nursing practice.

Key ideas or concepts in Orem's general theory of nursing are often referred to under three inter-related sub-headings, namely: her theory of self care; her theory of self care deficit(s) and her theory of nursing systems. For Orem, self-care is concerned with those activities that individuals engage in, on their own behalf, which are geared towards the maintenance of their life, health and well-being. For Orem, self-care agency is, obviously, closely connected to self-care and more specifically, refers to the individual's ability to engage in self-care. Orem makes further qualifying remarks whereby she states that an individual's self-care agency is heavily influenced by his/her age and associated stage (or phase) of developmental state; by his/her personal (and unique) life experiences; his/her particular socio-cultural background (and subsequent 'orientation'); and also by his/her particular health status and the personal physical and meta-physical resources available to the person at any given time. For Orem, therapeutic self-care demand refers to the combination of all self-care actions that are to be engaged in as a means to meet self-care requisites, and, importantly, Orem identifies three types (or categories) of self-care requisites: universal, developmental and health deviation.

For Orem, universal self-care requisites are those synonymous with the maintenance of the integrity of human structure and functioning and

Table 8.1. Orem's universal self-care requisites

- The maintenance of a sufficient intake of air
- The maintenance of a sufficient intake of water
- The maintenance of a sufficient intake of food
- The provision of care associated with elimination processes and excrements
- The maintenance of a balance between activity and rest
- The maintenance of a balance between solitude and social interaction
- The prevention of hazards to human life, human functioning and human well-being
- The promotion of human functioning and development within social groups in accordance with human potential, known human limitations, and the human desire to be 'normal' (Sometimes referred to as promoting 'normalcy')

From Orem, 1980: 42

are common to every human (these are listed in *Table 8.1* and expanded upon in *Table 8.2*) and perhaps not surprisingly, serve as the framework for assessment. Developmental self-care requisites, Orem declares, are those associated with individual developmental processes; they are holistic in that the developmental 'challenge' can occur in any of the dimensions of the person. For example, a psychological/intellectual challenge associated with one's teenage years, a physiological development of adjusting to gradual physical deterioration (e.g. having to start to wear glasses or wear a hearing aid), or a social development as one moves into a new peer group or moves to a new town. Health deviations of self-care are those associated with or those required in changes to one's holistic well-being or condition as a result of illness, injury, or disease.

Although the original ideas of the model were expressed prior to Kuhn's (1962) classic work on meta-paradigms, the original 1971 edition of her book speaks clearly to each of the four Khunian meta-paradigms of person, health, nursing and environment, albeit implicitly in some cases, and she says more about some meta-paradigms than she does about others.

Nursing

Given the centrality of the concept of self-care to Orem's model of nursing, readers will not be taken aback by the causality Orem posits between nursing and self-care. Indeed she asserts that nursing is required when the person has a self-care deficit. Orem (1980: 7) expresses this idea in the following way:

Nursing is required whenever the maintenance of continuous self-care requires the use of special techniques and the application of scientific knowledge in providing care or in designing it.

Self-care deficits occur when a person's capacity or capability to meet the need is 'out-stripped' by the self-care demand. In other words, the demand is greater than the person's self-care ability.

With some attention-grabbing and atypical statements, Orem (1980) draws attention to the fact that nursing, perhaps ironically, is not made or produced by nurses. For Orem, nursing can only occur when there is a need for nursing and an ability to provide nursing. She predicates that nursing then is a service, a mode of helping human beings and not a tangible commodity. Orem (1980: 5) continues, contending that:

Nursing's form or structure is derived from actions deliberately selected and performed by nurses to help individuals or groups under their care to maintain or change conditions in themselves or their environment.

With the essential and required interpersonal context for nursing established, Orem (1980) continues to purport that, given this context, a contract or agreement between the nurse and patient (or his/her representative) is necessary or required for nursing to occur. Importantly, Orem (1980) is adamant that nursing involves action, indeed she states that nursing is action. Furthermore, while in no way demeaning the work of our medical colleagues, Orem (1980) is unyielding in drawing attention to the fundamental differences between nursing care and medical care (important differences that continue to be eroded by contemporary 'developments' in nursing such as nurse prescribing and nurse practitioners). Indeed Orem (1980: 14) offers some unwavering (and, maybe for some, contentious) statements regarding nursing's inappropriate conflation with and over-reliance on medicine when she declares that this reliance (and its associated physicians' orders) places nurses and the clients they work with in dire straits.

Orem (1980: 7) describes five areas of nursing practice:

- Area 1: Entering into and maintaining nurse–patient relationships with individuals, families or groups.
- Area 2: Determining if and how patients can be helped through nursing.
- Area 3: Responding to patients' requests, desires and needs for nurse contacts and assistance.
- Area 4: Prescribing, providing, and regulating direct help to patients (and their significant others) in the form of nursing.
- Area 5: Co-ordinating and integrating nursing with the patient's daily

living, other healthcare needed or being received, and social and educational services needed or being received.

Having outlined her views on the areas of nursing practice, Orem (1980) goes on to outline four goals of nursing, and these are all (not surprisingly) linked to the notion of self-care needs. For Orem nursing involves either/or/and:

- Goal 1: Reducing the self-care demand to an extent that the person can meet the demand independently.
- Goal 2: Increasing the self-care ability/capacity of the person so that the person can meet the demand independently.
- Goal 3: Equipping the significant others in providing care for the person when he/she is incapable of meeting the self-care demand independently.
- Goal 4: The nurse meeting the person's self-care demand directly.

Health

Orem (1980: 118) asserts that,

Health is a term that has considerable general utility in describing the state of wholeness or integrity of human beings.

Individuals, Orem continues, make their own judgements about whether or not they consider themselves healthy or unhealthy, and thus individuals then have their own ideas about what constitutes their own healthy (or unhealthy) state. Orem (1980: 118) differentiates between what she terms 'temporary indispositions', 'having a brief illness' and 'being injured' from those structural and/or functional changes that seriously interfere with human functioning, and she draws on the example of a child with a fracture of an extremity to illustrate this point. (In the view of the authors, here is evidence of a somewhat dated idea of what constitutes health/ill-health. Contemporary understanding and theories – see Rolland and others, 1994, in Nolan et al's book, 1996 – of even the most severe and chronic illnesses indicates that suffers will still often, after a period of adaptation and adjustment, describe themselves as healthy. Although it is fair to point out that perhaps Orem, 1980: 119, accounts for potential evolution in the views of health when she states that 'the meaning of the term health changes as views about people's human and biological characteristics change'.) Nevertheless, Orem (1980: 118) does qualify her views with her statement that,

Any deviation from normal structure or functioning is properly referred to as an absence of health in the sense of wholeness or integrity.

Orem (1980 is adamant that expressions of human health must include aspects of what she refers to as mental life, physiological and psychophysiological mechanisms and their physical (biological) structure, in addition to the person's interpersonal and social life. For Orem then, health is very much an integrated, holistic concept. Orem (1980) also offers some enlightened and advanced statements concerning health suggesting that,

> *Health is the responsibility of a society and its individual members and not of any one segment of that society.*

Perhaps with an indirect reference to certain humanistic philosophies, Orem (1980) argues that ill-health can, paradoxically, be 'good for' the individual; that ill-health or other human suffering can also bring individuals an increased understanding of themselves and others. Furthermore, significant and highly valuable personal qualities, such as courage, patience and altruism, can be developed and revealed as a result of the experience of personal ill-health and/or suffering.

Persons

Orem (1980) writes of persons as unitary sentient beings who are capable of making choices and pursuing goals, and that all people share the same universal self-care needs; how they go about meeting those universal needs, however, varies considerably from person to person. Orem (1980: 6) declares that in modern society, adults are expected to be self-reliant and responsible for themselves and for the well-being of their dependants. Given the centrality of the concept of self-care to Orem's nursing model, it should not be surprising that she posits self-care as a requirement of every human being, irrespective of age or gender. Accordingly, for Orem, to be human is to have a need for self-care. Interestingly though, while Orem points out that for people, self-care is voluntary (i.e. a person can choose not to engage in self-care), she maintains that it is a right and responsibility for people to engage in self-care in order to maintain their health, life and well-being. As a result, for Orem, it can be seen that not to engage in self-care is to renege on one's personal responsibility as a person. Orem also purports however that people need to learn how to engage in self-care; that self-care is acquired through social and intellectual experiences; through one's interpersonal relationships and culture. So there seems to be an unspoken, yet critical element of Orem's views of person here, namely, that to be a responsible human is to 'pass on' or help others learn about the centrality and importance of self-care.

Orem (1980) also purports that persons have consciousness, awareness, and thus sentience; they have the ability to think, feel and to know. For

Orem, people can use this sentience to enable them to make self-determined actions; that a person is capable of deliberating (to paraphrase) on a course of action even when he/she feels drawn in a different direction. Accordingly, Orem argues that people who take action to provide their own self-care or care for dependants have specialised capabilities for action (Orem, 1980).

Environment

Orem (1980) offers some specific statements about how the nurse can and should provide an environment that promotes the development of the person. In Orem's (1980: 66) words, providing a developmental environment requires the nurse to,

Provide or help to provide environmental conditions that motivate the person being helped to establish appropriate goals and adjust behaviour to achieve results specified by goals.

As with many other nursing models, Orem says less about the 'nursing' of the environment than she does about the other meta-paradigms. However, she does declare that the environment refers to all aspects, interpersonal, psychosocial and physical, and that all these elements need to be considered and adjusted in order to encourage development. Accordingly, Orem (1980: 66) declares that the essence of this domain of nursing is,

The continued and proper relating of selected environmental elements in light of the patient's special needs and the changes being sought in the patient's health state or manner of living.

Orem (1980) qualifies her remarks regarding the need for the adjustment of the environment by drawing attention to the relationship between the physical (external to the person) environment, and the person's psychosocial environment. While the astute reader may be able to see the strong influence of Nightingale's (1859) axiomatic view of nursing here (namely, that nurses do not heal anyone, but rather place the person in the best position to let nature heal them), and/or the impact of some developmental psychology maxims (most especially that the individual can be significantly affected by the particular physical and psychosocial environment that they encounter [Rogers, 1962]), it is still heartening to see a nursing model focus on more than the immediate physiological well-being and pay specific attention to the interactions between individuals and the environment they inhabit. It may be of interest to note that for Orem (1980: 67), the effectiveness of the nurse's methods of assistance in this area (i.e. nursing the environment) is highly dependent upon the nurse's creativity and his or her knowledge of and respect for people. This has major implications for nursing practice yet seldom does it appear or is it discussed within the nursing literature or nursing community. The implication is that creative nurses would look beyond the physical and psychological boundaries of the individual person needing nursing and will seek to explore creative ways to foster the most appropriate, developmentally conducive environment. Such nurses then seek to create the conditions under which individuals can best learn how to meet their own self-care demands.

Nursing systems and methods

Whereas some other nursing models refer to nursing roles, Orem (1980) speaks of nursing systems and methods, and she describes three types of nursing systems:

- Wholly compensatory system.
- Partially compensatory system.
- Supportive-educative (developmental) nursing system.

Orem (1980) declares that nurses can determine which system they are operating in by asking the question: Who can or should perform the person's self-care actions? If the answer is 'the nurse', the wholly compensatory system is required. If the answer is that the person can perform some, but not all self-care actions him or herself, then the partially compensatory system is required. If the answer is the person him or herself, then the partially compensatory system is required. (The authors would advance Orem's (1980) position here; namely that the nurse can operate in more than one system simultaneously with the same person. It is the nature of the particular problem and the extent of the self-care deficit(s) that govern the resultant nursing system. For example, a person with a broken leg may need assistance with some universal self-care deficits (e.g. partially compensatory) but would only require support and education (supportive-educative system) regarding passive physiotherapy.) Orem (1980) also illustrates how the nurse and client will often move between these different systems as care progresses or regresses. What is perhaps alluded to by Orem (1980), yet the authors would argue could be made more clear, is the perpetual attempt to return the client to his or her maximum level of self-care agency and with that, a persistent effort to move from actions in the wholly compensatory system to actions in the supportive-educative system.

Having identified these overarching systems, Orem (1980) proceeds to identify five nursing methods of helping, namely:

- Doing for or acting for another.
- Guiding and directing another.
- Providing physical support.
- Providing psychological support.
- Providing an environment that supports development.

Examination of these systems indicates that some are clearly more (perhaps only) applicable to some methods more than others (and vice versa). For example, the nursing method 'acting for/doing for the patient' has a high degree of congruence with the system 'totally compensatory/supportive' and is difficult to reconcile with the system 'teaching/supporting'. As a result, when care is being planned for a client when using Orem's model, it may be prudent for the nurse to include in the client's plan of care which nursing method(s) of help are being used to meet the particular goal.

Clinical application of Orem's model

Our examination of the extant literature that focuses on Orem's model indicates that attempts have been made to apply this model in a variety of nursing situations and specialty areas (see below). In addition, our review showed that when compared to other nursing models, Orem's model has arguably a more developed body of associated literature. One consequence of this larger body of work is that it is more difficult to identify one key author who has advanced the knowledge base more than any other (apart from Orem's own revisited versions of her model). As a result, for our principal example of the clinical application of Orem's model, while we understandably draw heavily on Orem's own examples and explanations, we also use elements of other existing work (for example Taylor, 1988; Aggleton and Chalmers, 2000; Martinez, 2005). We follow this with a brief review of other literature which has attempted to apply and/or operationalise Orem's model in a variety of clinical/empirical ways.

Aggleton and Chalmers (2000) rightly point out that the term 'assessment' is not used with much frequency in Orem's work; instead she refers to nurses obtaining a 'nursing history'. Nevertheless, taking a nursing history or assessment is focused on determining whether or not the person has a self-care deficit; and this is done by examining the person's universal, developmental and health deviation self-care requisites. Earlier Pearson and Vaughan (1986) had made very similar arguments, suggesting that from the self-care perspective, assessment focuses on the three categories of self-care requisites and self-care deficits. Accordingly, our nursing history (assessment) will use such a format. It is important to note (and here the authors wholeheartedly applaud the logic and reasoning of

Table 8.2. General sets of actions for meeting the eight universal self-care requisites

The maintenance of a sufficient intake of air, water and food
- Taking in that quantity required for normal functioning with adjustments for internal and external factors that can affect the requirement
- Preserving the integrity of the associated anatomical structures and physiological processes
- Enjoy the pleasurable experiences of breathing, drinking and eating without abuses

The provision of care associated with elimination processes and excrements.
- Bringing about and maintaining internal and external conditions necessary for the regulation of eliminative processes
- Managing the process of elimination (including protection of the structures and processes involved) and disposal of excrements
- Providing subsequent hygienic care of body surfaces and parts
- Caring for the environment as needed to maintain sanitary conditions

Maintenance of a balance between activity and rest
- Selecting activities that stimulate, engage, and keep in balance physical movement, affective responses, intellectual effort and social interaction
- Recognising and attending to manifestations of needs for rest and activity
- Using personal capabilities, interests and values as well as culturally prescribed norms as bases for development of a rest–activity pattern

Maintenance of a balance between solitude and social interaction
- Maintaining that quality and balance necessary for the development of personal autonomy and enduring social relations that foster effective functioning of individuals
- Fostering bonds of affection, love, friendship and friendship; effectively managing impulses to use others for selfish purposes, disregarding their individuality, integrity and rights
- Providing conditions of social warmth and closeness essential for continuing development and adjustment
- Promoting individual autonomy as well as group membership

Prevention of hazards to life, functioning and well-being
- Being alert to types of hazards that are likely to occur
- Taking action to prevent the occurrence of events that may lead to the development of hazardous situations
- Removing or protecting oneself from hazardous situations when a hazard cannot be eliminated
- Controlling hazardous situations to eliminate danger to life or well-being

Promotion of normalcy
- Developing and maintaining a realistic self-concept
- Taking action to foster specific human developments
- Taking action to maintain and promote the integrity of one's human structure and functioning
- Identifying and attending to deviations from one's structural and functional norms

Adapted from Orem, 1980

this clinical decision; all too often volume and pure quantity of information is mistaken for parsimonious, accurate and relevant information gathered during the assessment) that Orem maintains that nurses should not gather large amounts of irrelevant data during the assessment but instead should tailor the taking of a nursing history to the needs of the individual patient. It is also critical to note that Orem (1980) emphasises that nurses need to observe, measure and have dialogue during the assessment; that it is by engaging in these actions that the assessing nurse can gather the relevant assessment data and information.

For our clinical case example, we have drawn on a real client, although all details and data pertaining to the person have been changed in order to maintain his (or her) complete confidentiality.

Case example

Dale is a 17-year-old adolescent male who has presented himself at the Accident and Emergency department (Emergency Room for North America readership). Dale explains to the assessing nurse that he has taken an overdose of antidepressant medication imipramine (a mild tricyclic). He claims that he was intending to kill himself, although he states that he did not take more than six tablets before he decided to stop and make his way to the Accident and Emergency department and that this occurred approximately 25 minutes before Dale showed up at the hospital. Several old and more recent superficial scars are evident on both of his wrists/forearms.

Nursing assessment (history) on presentation at accident and emergency

Universal self-care requisites

- The maintenance of a sufficient intake of air, water and food

Is the client taking in that quantity required for normal functioning?
Air: Yes, no evidence of hypoxia, dyspneoa, or cyanosis. Client appears to be breathing regularly and deeply.

Water: Yes, no evidence of dehydration or over-hydration. Mucus membranes appear moist, no reports of excessive thirst, although client does say he wants a drink. Passed urine without pain or difficulty.

Food: Yes, no evidence of malnourishment, client weighs 86.2 kg and his 1.73 m tall. Says he does not feel hungry.

There is no evidence to suggest that there has been any change to the integrity of the associated anatomical structures; chest and abdominal X-rays show nothing of concern. No physical external or internal trauma evident. No signs or symptoms of any disruption to the client's physiological processes of respiration, hydration and ingestion, e.g bowel sounds normal and active, breath sounds in each lobe of the lungs, blood pressure and pulse rate within normal limits for a 17-year-old man.

There may be some evidence to suggest that the client does not currently enjoy the pleasurable experiences of eating and drinking. The client reports that, at times, he does not have a 'healthy appetite' (although there is no evidence that he is underweight). He claims he has lost 9 kg in weight over the last month.

- The provision of care associated with elimination processes and excrements

Is the client maintaining the internal and external conditions necessary for the regulation of eliminative processes?

Yes: Client reports that he has had no problems with his bowels and had his bowels open yesterday. No pain or discomfort when passing urine or faeces. No evidence of deterioration in tissue integrity evident in the client's groin or perineal area.

- Maintenance of a balance between activity and rest

Is the client selecting activities that stimulate, engage, and keep in balance physical movement, affective responses, intellectual effort and social interaction?

No: The client reports that he seldom engages in any form of physical exercise, often spends the majority of his time alone in his room. He spends most of his time 'interacting' in a virtual environment through mediums such as 'Face Book' and 'My Space'. His affective responses appear to be a significant problem and suggest the presence of a self-care deficit. For instance, Dale says that he has great difficulty talking about his problems with anyone and yet he also says that his self-esteem and perception of self-worth are both low right now. He is, however, unwilling or unable to discuss these feelings with any of his friends or family and accordingly, his affective responses are stilted. Similarly, his social interactions appear to be mostly restricted to his 'virtual' contacts and 'online' friends. As a result, he seldom interacts face-to-face with his friends and peers.

Does the client recognise and attend to manifestations of needs for rest and activity?

There may be a self-care deficit here. There is no evidence that the client has difficulty resting (physically). He says that at times he has difficulty sleeping yet he also reports that he often stays in bed until quite late in the morning (when he does not have to go to school). If anything, as Dale describes his weekly and daily activities, it is more the case that he is underactive and that he might benefit from engaging is more physical activity (particularly given the well-documented antidepressant effects of moderate exercise programmes).

Does the client appear to use personal capabilities, interests and values as well as culturally prescribed norms as bases for the development of a rest–activity pattern?

Dale describes his 'social scene' as one that primarily revolves around virtual or 'web-based' interactions with his friends; this is a cultural norm for both Dale and his peer group. As a result, yes, Dale does appear to be using some of his personal capabilities, interests and values as an influence on his patterns of activity/rest.

- Maintenance of a balance between solitude and social interaction

Does the client maintain that quality and balance necessary for the development of personal autonomy and enduring social relations that foster effective functioning of individuals?

No: There may be a self-care deficit here. As described in the previous area of assessment, Dale describes his 'social scene' as one that primarily revolves around virtual or 'web-based' interactions with his friends; accordingly this is a cultural norm for both Dale and his peer group. Solitude and social interaction are thus arguably encountered and experienced differently for young people belonging to 'generation X' since their social interaction often occurs when they are simultaneously isolated (i.e. sat at their computer, logged on). It is difficult to reconcile Dale's expressions of low self-esteem and low mood with ideas around enduring social relationships. It is possible that the virtual and online relationships he is engaged in are not sufficiently or adequately fostering his own effective functioning.

Has the client fostered bonds of affection, love and friendship; effectively managing impulses to use others for selfish purposes, disregarding their individuality, integrity and rights?

No: There appears to be evidence of a self-care deficit here. Dale states that he has very few close friends and has trouble 'fitting in' with his peer group. He reports that he is not very close to his family (as he and his mother do not 'get on'). As a result it is possible that Dale has a self-care deficit in terms of his need for love and affection. This would then very likely have a profound effect on his self-esteem and self-worth.

Does the client report experiencing the conditions of social warmth and closeness essential for continuing development and adjustment?

No: As stated above, there is evidence to indicate the presence of a self-care deficit here. Dale states that he seldom experiences a strong sense of acceptance from his peer group, he has very few close friends, and reports that he is not very close to his family. As a result it is difficult to see where Dale has been experiencing any strong sense of social warmth and interpersonal closeness. Consequently and particularly given his particular stage of life, it is possible (probable) that this absence of experiences will affect his development and adjustment.

Is there evidence of activities to promote individual autonomy as well as group membership?

At this moment in time, while there is little evidence to suggest that Dale's individual autonomy is well developed, he reports that most of his concerns appear to centre on group/peer membership and acceptance.

- Prevention of hazards to life, functioning and well-being

Does the client appear to be alert to types of hazards that are likely to occur?

No: From what Dale has reported, he does not appear to have fully understood the link between his apparent lack of acceptance, closeness and social warmth, his subsequent low self-esteem and low self-worth and the episodes of self-harm.

Does the client appear to take action to prevent the occurrence of events that may lead to the development of hazardous situations?

In terms of the hazardous situation that the client presents with, namely, repeated episodes of self-harm, there is little evidence that Dale is taking action to prevent those from occurring.

Has the client removed or protected himself from hazardous situations when a hazard cannot be eliminated?

No: Dale still makes frequent attempts to engage with and subsequently gain acceptance from his peer group.

- Promotion of normalcy

Does the client appear to be developing and maintaining a realistic self-concept?

No: This a key development aspect for Dale (given his age).

Does the client appear to be taking action to foster specific human developments?

To some extent but more is needed. Given that he has significant development tasks and challenges at the moment, this is where much of his attention and focus might be directed.

Does the client appear to be taking action to maintain and promote the integrity of his human structure and functioning?

No: As stated above there is compelling evidence that some of Dale's actions are directed at harming his human structure.

Does the client appear to be identifying and attending to deviations from his structural and functional norms?

No

Developmental self-care requisites

Orem (1980: 47) refers to developmental self-care deficits as specialised expressions of universal self-care requisites. In Dale's case, his developmental self-care requisites focus on those associated with late adolescence. There exists a very well-developed literature on the developmental tasks facing adolescents (see for examples, Carnegie Council on Adolescent Development, 1995; Cobb, 1994; Dryfoos, 1990; Erikson, 1968; Nightingale and Wolverton, 1993). While acknowledging some scope for individual variation, it has been argued that the principal development mission that adolescents face is to create their established identity and become complete and productive adults. In order to achieve this, additional developmental tasks often include: achieving emotional independence from parents and other adults; establishing new and more mature relations with both genders in their age group; achieving an understanding of what it means to be a man or a woman; acceptance of one's body; preparing for adult life (e.g. career, economic stability, long-term relationships, having one's own family); developing a personal ideology and aspiring to/achieving socially responsible behaviour.

In Dale's case there is evidence that he may have a self-care deficit with regards to the task/dynamic of 'separation versus individualism'; of achieving emotional independence from parents. Indeed, it is not the issue of separation from parents and more a matter of experiencing love and acceptance. Indeed, the value that Dale places on the acceptance from his peer group may well have added significance given that he reports how he gets little of this from his parents. This then affects the nature of the relationships he seeks from his peer group, perhaps making them more akin

Table 8.3. Planning of nursing intervention for client who presented at accident and emergency (emergency room)

Prevention of hazards to life, functioning and well-being
Problem
- Dale has ingested a relatively small overdose of imipramine (a tricyclic antidepressant which, while low risk, should still be regarded as serious and potentially fatal in children
Goal/aim
- Ensure and maintain Dale's physical integrity and safety.
Intervention/rationale
- Administer emetic agent (Ipecac) as per physician's order and monitor effects
- Monitor/record vital signs every 15 minutes and notify Physician if any major changes occur
- Pay particular attention to and observe for signs of tachycardia, widened QRS complex via ECG reading and any neurological disturbances as these are the most common side-effects of over-dose with tricyclic antidepressant medication (BMA/RPSGB, 2009)
Nursing actions
- Acting for/totally compensatory

Promotion of normalcy
Problem
- Dale appears to have low self-esteem, low-self worth, and a significant need for acceptance and 'love' (perhaps exacerbated by the limited relationship he has with his parental figures)
- Dale appears to be struggling with discovering his place in the world (his world view) and of what it means to be an adult male. (appropriately for his age/stage of development)

Goal/aim
- Begin to improve Dale's self-esteem and acceptance of himself; as evidenced by noting some use by Dale of positive self-statements, less frequent use of negative self-expressions. Consider using repeated measures on a hope/hopelessness scale
Intervention/rationale
- Provide a supportive, accepting, non-judgemental environment
- Communicate to Dale that he matters, that you care about his well-being and situation
- Offer time and space for Dale to speak about what he has been experiencing and allow any ventilation of emotions/feelings
- Ask him 'Where does it hurt?' (psychologically)

- Offer reassurance and support that the behaviours Dale has engaged in are not uncommon (especially in his age group), nor do they indicate that he is 'mad' or 'abnormal'
- Encourage Dale to reflect on what needs he is having met through or by engaging with his 'virtual' or 'online' peer group
- Encourage Dale to explore and consider possible alternative ways that these needs might be met
- While offering guidance and suggestions towards how these needs might be met, it would be prudent to remind Dale that you will respect whatever decision he makes, that he has 'room' and the responsibility for his own decisions, and that he will be accountable for the consequences of those decisions
- Encourage Dale to reflect on and think about where and who he might go to in order to receive continuing expressions of warmth and love (e.g. he says he gets on very well with his uncle)
- Encourage Dale to think about alternative ways of coping (that do not involve self-harming) when he feels or experiences low self-esteem/worth, rejection from his loved ones and/or peer group

Nursing actions
- Supporting the client.
- Providing an (interpersonal) environment in which the client can develop and grow.
- Guiding the client

Maintenance of a balance between solitude and social interaction

Problem
- Dale appears to need to establish new and more mature relations with both genders in their age group

Goal/aim
- Gain formal agreement from Dale that he will attempt to form a new relationship with someone outside of his current peer group.

Intervention/rationale
- Encourage Dale to explore additional possible social situations and groups that he might join (e.g. Dale says he enjoys music and there are several music groups locally)
- Provide support and encouragement for him to attend one of these new meetings 'of interest' within one week of discharge

Nursing actions
- Supporting the client.
- Providing an (interpersonal) environment in which the client can develop and grow
- Guiding the client

to parent-to-child relationships (*à la* Berne, 1962) and less 'mature'. There is no evidence that he has a problem with accepting his body per se, although he does not appear to have fully accepted himself. It is no surprise that he has difficulty accepting himself since, according to Dale, this message of acceptance was not consistently provided by his parents and thus he has internalised these perceptions for himself. As a result, there is evidence of a self-care deficit in terms of Dale discovering his place in the world (his world view) and of what it means to be an adult male.

Health deviation self-care requisites

There is no evidence that Dale is experiencing any deficits related to health-deviation self-care requisites other than the need to stabilise him physically and ensure his physical longevity is not under threat. Dale has no evidence of any specific forms of pathology, illness or disability.

Testing and/or evaluating Orem's model in clinical practice

Various, usually small-scale studies, and a few discursive papers have focused on examining/determining the effectiveness of Orem's model (or parts thereof) in clinical practice. Relatively early work undertaken by Hanucharurnkui and Vinya-nguag (1991) attempted to test the value of clients who engage in self-care post-operatively. Having provided the experimental group with a number of instruction activities that would (theoretically) increase their self-care agency (e.g. how to perform deep breathing and limb movement exercises), participants' rate of recovery (measured by means of various instruments) was then compared to a control group. The findings strongly suggested that engaging in a variety of self-care activities post-operatively significantly shortened their post-operative hospitalisation and increased their overall level of satisfaction. Aish and Isenberg's (1996) study of nutritional self-care following a myocardial infarction produced similar findings. After providing the experimental group with an intervention geared towards lowering animal fat in their diets (and thus improving their nutritional self-care agency), significant differences were found between the control and experimental groups with respect to intake of fat. Interestingly, no significant differences were found between the groups with respect to their self-care agency scores.

Hart (1995) attempted to examine a causal model of relationships between self-care agency, basic prenatal decisions, foundations for dependent-care agency and selected pregnancy outcomes. With a sample size of 127 pregnant women, Hart's findings suggested that increased self-care agency had a direct (positive) effect on basic prenatal care actions and foundations for dependent-care agency. Hart (1995) concluded that these findings lend further empirical support for (aspects of) Orem's (1980) model. Hart and Foster's (1998) follow up, secondary analysis study of pregnant women found that participants who enrolled into childbirth education classes had higher self-care agency scores.

A similar retrospective test of (elements of) Orem's (1980) model was undertaken by Gaffney and Moore (1996), who chose to test the relationship between maternal dependent care performance and Orem's basic conditioning factors (e.g. age, ethnic group, socio-economic status, maternal employment, etc.). From a convenience sample of 380 participants, only some support for the hypothesis was found; that is 13% of the variance in the mothers' dependent care performance could be explained by differences in these so-called basic conditioning factors. Mosher and Moore (1998) likewise wished to examine the relationships between self-concept and self-care, dependent care and basic conditioning factors. Drawing on a sample of 74 children with cancer, some evidence was found which suggested that when the children had higher self-concept scores they engaged in more self-care activities and yet also received more dependent care from their mothers.

Soderhamn and Cliffordson's (2001) study of the structure of self-care in older Swedish adults provided support for Orem's postulated relationship between self-care agency and self-care demand. Their results indicated that when self-care demand is balanced by the presence/influence of five conditioning factors, it is significantly and positively balanced with self-care agency.

Case studies

Taylor (1988) draws on a clinical example as an attempt to apply Orem's (1980) model, and especially the key ideas around self-care deficits to an individual diagnosed and living with amyotrophic lateral sclerosis. (ALS, commonly referred to as Lou Gehrig's disease in North America, is a progressive, degenerative disease of the motor neurons and in most cases results in fatality.) Taylor's paper provides a reasonable example of how assessment (or nursing history taking) can be focused on the client's ability to self-care versus the self-care demands he is facing. It may be no coincidence that a person living with a chronic and degenerative neurological disease was chosen, as such individuals present with many self-care deficits and yet no acute, life-threatening problems. The case study focuses far more on the physiological, and, to a lesser extent, social aspects of the self-care requisites and not enough attention or detail is paid to the psychological self-care requisites. For example, as the disease progresses and the client's self-care agency further diminishes, he will require more and more 'totally compensatory nursing actions' and this needs to be taken into account when considering his balance between solitude and social interaction. Furthermore, with respect to the universal self-care demands related to 'promotion of normalcy'; coming to terms with chronic, seriously debilitating illness; the loss of major roles (e.g. 'family breadwinner'); becoming increasingly dependent upon others; the increasing loss of dignity; and, not least, the fear/anxiety about his impending death, were almost completely absent from the paper. (Such focus and emphasis on the physiological components of nursing, when drawing on many nursing models, is, the authors have found, very common and highlights a significant gap in the associated literature.)

Martinez (2005) offers a similar paper to Taylor although she focuses on self-care for stoma surgery rather than a chronic, degenerative illness. Martinez (2005) illustrates the three stage process she undertook: Firstly assessing the client's self-care agency and self-care demands, secondly the selection of particular and effective interventions geared to promote the client's self-care agency, and thirdly, the so-called production of and management of nursing systems which, for Martinez (2005), occurred when she interacted with the client and engaged in re-assessment, re-implementation and re-evaluation. To her credit, Martinez (2005) does include attention to 'psychological' dimensions and highlighted post-surgical anxiety as the first priority diagnosis and alterations in body image as the second. While the authors applaud such attention, the paper lacked detail in how Orem's model was applied to this client. For example, which specific self-care deficit(s) did post-surgical anxiety refer to? And should not alterations to body image have been located within the 'promotion of normalcy' self-care requisite? Nevertheless, the focus on non-physiological aspects of the person does demonstrate the potential width of application and utility of Orem's model.

Practice development papers based on Orem's model

A number of papers have been produced that report various practice development initiatives in nursing, each of which was guided by Orem's model, or used it as the underpinning theory for development. These initiatives have occurred in a range of different clinical settings/scenarios including medication discharge planning in a general hospital (Schneider et al, 1993), a supportive/educative programme for clients with advanced heart failure (Jaarsma et al, 1998), and an education programme in oncology for clients with low literacy skills (Wilson et al, 2003). For the medication discharge planning programme, Schneider et al (1993) made the argument that clients who implement better self-care while at home are less likely to be re-admitted to hospital, and they argued that re-admissions might then be one measure of enacting self-care. While the sample size of 54 participants does not enable firm conclusions to be drawn, the results from this paper indicate that hospital re-admissions were reduced for the participants who received the medication discharge planning; that re-admissions were reduced for those with greater self-care agency.

Jaarsma et al (1997) argued that clients with heart failure (and their families) face significant and changing self-care demands as a consequence of experiencing the disease and its associated treatment. Accordingly, they designed an assessment tool for the accurate determination of the self-care demand and an educative/supportive programme designed to increase the client's self-care agency (mostly via Orem's 1980 nursing roles of teaching and guiding) with particular reference to the challenges associated with advanced heart failure. Unfortunately, no data were made available pertaining to the testing of this educative/supportive programme.

Wilson et al (2003) used Orem's model to examine clients' self-care agency with respect to reading, comprehension, reasoning, perception and so-called verbal skills. Acquiring this assessment information then allowed the development of appropriately designed client education materials (especially for those with low literacy skills). Focusing initially within oncology, information cards relating to treatment side effects associated with radiation therapy were designed and distributed to a sample of 238 clients. Measures of client comprehension of these cards were then taken and the results showed that these cards were less then ideal as a teaching tool for clients with cancer who have limited reading and comprehension skills.

Empirical papers that use Orem's model as the theoretical underpinning

Several papers have been published which report empirical research studies that used Orem's model as the underpinning theoretical framework. Pickens (1999) reports on a qualitative study of the desire for 'normalcy' as narrated by six men and 13 women. Not only does this paper use Orem's (1980) model as the underpinning theoretical framework but the study also focuses on achieving one of Orem's universal self-care requisites. The participants described categories of 'desire for normalcy', namely, having normal things and experiences, doing meaningful activities, and being well, safe, free and independent. Similarly, Zrinyi and Zekanya (2001) report the findings from a study which aimed to determine whether or not clients' self-care agency improved between the time of being admitted to hospital and subsequent discharge. In other words, the study can be regarded as examining if the care provided enhances the clients' independence (self-care agency). Drawing on a convenience sample of 162 clients from a mixture of wards/units (e.g. internal medicine, oncology, gynaecology, medical-surgical), self-care agency scores showed no significant change between admission and discharge. In conclusion, the authors raise a number of very interesting and worthwhile questions concerning whether or not acute care settings/ facilities are appropriate points of intervention to improve self-care capabilities. A more recent qualitative study was carried out by Moore and Beckwith (2006) who wished to explore and determine what self-care and dependent care activities children with cancer and their parents engaged in as a means to meet their self-care requisites. A purposeful sample of nine children with cancer and 18 parents provided data which, when analysed, indicated that a range of self-care operations (e.g. estimative, transitional and productive) were used to meet the self-care requisites. Also Dalton et al (2006) designed an evaluation study of a diabetes management home care programme based upon Orem's (1980) model. Three groups of clients with diabetes were obtained with two groups receiving an experimental diabetes disease management programme. Various measures were undertaken and no statistically significant findings were found between the groups.

A very interesting and thoughtful study was undertaken by McDermott (1993) who wished to test the relationship between Orem's (1980) concept of self-care agency and learned helplessness (albeit in a slightly adapted form from Seligman's original 1975 theory). The author accessed a convenience sample of 309 volunteers ('healthy' men and women) and, perhaps not surprisingly, the proposed null-hypothesis was supported. To paraphrase, the less helpless a person felt, the greater his/her score was on a self-care agency scale. Campbell and Weber (2000) based their test of a model of women's responses to battering on Orem's (1980) concept of self-care. The authors hypothesised that age, educational level and cultural influences would all be directly related to relational conflict (which in turn would be negatively related to self-care agency). In a convenience sample of 117 women, only a borderline fit for their model was found. Geden and Taylor (1999) undertook a descriptive study that focused on the collaborative care systems of couples and used Orem's (1980) model as the underpinning theoretical framework. The data obtained from 108 couples showed some support (27%) for the relationship between certain variables and the extent of collaborative care; to paraphrase, a small number of the couples had higher collaborative care scores if they had higher cohesion in the family. Cox and Taylor's (2005)paper is less akin to an empirical study and more of a review of published literature, nevertheless the authors still used Orem's model as 'the theoretical approach for examining current scientific evidence about children with asthma'. Unfortunately, Cox and Taylor (2005) do not indicate how they identified the literature to include in the review, nor did they provide inclusion/exclusion criteria or even the total number of papers reviewed. As a result, their 'findings' should be regarded with a degree of caution.

Suggested further reading: Theoretical comparisons and explorations of Orem's model

- Taylor (1991): This is a descriptive and somewhat discursive paper that offers a structural model to guide nursing diagnosis, based on Orem's model.
- Bliss-Holtz (1996): This discursive paper focuses on decision-making processes, based on Orem's model, which then produce diagnostic statements concerning the person's self-care agency/self-care demand.
- Fawdry et al (1996): This is a theoretical paper that attempts to explore intergenerational nursing systems from three perspectives, including Orem's dependent care.
- de Montigny et al (1997): This article explains how Orem's model (and Roy's model – see *Chapter 6*) is used as the underpinning framework for teaching family nursing theory/practice.
- McQuiston and Campbell (1997): This paper makes the case for theoretical substruction as a guide for theory testing research that draws on two propositions from Orem's model; basic conditioning factors and self-care agency.
- Walker and Grobe (1999): This is a theoretical discussion paper that attempts to explore the conceptual composition of thriving, suggesting that thriving is made up of the concepts of integration of nutrition, and psychosocial and lifestyle concerns. The authors then attempt to situate this exploration in the broader context of Orem's model.
- Moore and Pichler (2000): This paper is a literature review of published research on basic conditioning factors (*à la* Orem's model).
- Arndt and Horodynski (2004): This paper explores concepts contained within Orem's model, including: dependent-care and educative-supportive nursing systems. These are explored within the context of a project focusing on nutrition in toddlers.
- Allison (2007): This interesting article explores in detail the meaning of Orem's universal self-care requisite 'balance between activity and rest'. The paper advances a thorough understanding of this self-care requisite and offers some potential clinical applications of this increased understanding (e.g. it offers a guide for a nursing clinical assessment and suggested nursing actions pertaining to this self-care requisite).

References

Aggleton P, Chalmers H (2000) *Nursing Models and Nursing Practice* 2nd edn. Macmillan Press, Basingstoke

Aish AE, Isenberg M (1996) Effects of Orem-based nursing intervention on nutritional self-care of myocardial infarction patients. *International Journal of Nursing Studies* **33**(3): 259–70

Allison SE (2007) Self-care requirements for activity and rest: An Orem nursing focus. *Nursing Science Quarterly* **20**(1): 68–76

Arndt MJ, Horodynski MAO (2004) Theory of dependent-care in research with parents with toddlers: the Neat project. *Nursing Science Quarterly* **17**(4): 345–50

Berne E (1962) *The Games People Play: The Psychology of Human Relationships.* Penguin, London

Bliss-Holtz J (1996) Using Orem's theory to generate nursing diagnoses for electronic documentation. *Nursing Science Quarterly* **9**(3): 121–5

BMA/RPSGB (2009) *British National Formulary.* British Medical Association/ Royal Pharmacological Society of Great Britain, London

Campbell JC, Weber N (2000) An empirical test of a self-care model of women's responses to battering. *Nursing Science Quarterly* **13**(1): 45–53

Carnegie Council on Adolescent Development (1995) *Great Transitions: Preparing Adolescents for a New Century.* Carnegie Corporation, New York

Cobb NJ (1994) *Adolescence: Continuity, Change, and Diversity.* Mayfield Publishing, Mountain View, Ca

Cox KR, Taylor SG (2005) Orem's self-care deficit nursing theory: Pediatric asthma as an exemplar. *Nursing Science Quarterly* **18**(3) 249–57

deMontigny F, Dumas L, Boldue L, Blais S (1997) Teaching family nursing based on conceptual models of nursing. *Journal of Advanced Nursing* **3**(3): 267–79

Dalton J, Garvey J, Samia LW (2006) Evaluation of a diabetes disease management home care program. *Home Health Care Management and Practice* **18**(4): 272–85

Dryfoos JG (1990) *Adolescents at Risk: Prevalence and Prevention.* Oxford University Press, New York

Erikson EH (1968) *Identity: Youth and Crisis.* WW Norton, New York

Fawdry MK, Berry ML, Rajacich D (1996) The articulation of nursing systems with dependent care systems of intergenerational caregivers. *Nursing Science Quarterly* **9**(1): 22–6

Gaffney K, Moore JB (1996) Testing Orem's theory of self-care deficit: Dependent care agent performance for children. *Nursing Science Quarterly* **9**(4): 160–4

Geden EA, Taylor SG (1999) Theoretical and empirical description of an adult couple's collaborative self-care system. *Nursing Science Quarterly* **12**(4): 329–34

Hanucharurnkui S, Vinya-nguag P (1991) Effects of promoting patients' participation in self-care on post-operative recovery and satisfaction with care. *Nursing Science Quarterly* **4**(1): 14–20

Hart MA (1995) Orem's self-care deficit theory: Research with pregnant women. *Nursing Science Quarterly* **8**(3): 120–6

Hart MA, Foster SN (1998) Self-care agency in two groups of pregnant women. *Nursing Science Quarterly* **11**(4): 167–71

Jaarsma T, Halferns R, Senten M, Abu Saad HH, Dracup K (1998) Developing a supportive education program for patients with advanced heart failure within Orem's general theory of nursing. *Nursing Science Quarterly* **11**(2): 79–85

Kuhn T (1962) *The Structure of Scientific Revolutions* 3rd edn. Chicago University Press, Chicago

McDermott MA (1993) Learned helplessness as an interacting variable with self-care agency: Testing a theoretical model. *Nursing Science Quarterly* **6**(1) 28–38

McKenna HP, Slevin OD (2008) *Nursing Models, Theories and Practice*. Blackwell Science, Oxford

McQuiston CM, Campbell JC (1997) Theoretical substruction: A guide for theory testing research. *Nursing Science Quarterly* **10**(3): 117–23

Martinez LA (2005) Self-care for stoma surgery: Mastering independent stoma self-care skills in an elderly woman. *Nursing Science Quarterly* **18**(1): 66–9

Maslow A (1954) *Motivation and Personality*. Harper Row, New York

Moore JB, Pichler VH (2000) Measurement of Orem's basic conditioning factors: A review of published research. *Nursing Science Quarterly* **13**(2): 137–42

Moore JB, Beckwith AE (2006) Self-care operations and nursing interventions for children with cancer and their patients. *Nursing Science Quarterly* **19**(2): 147–56

Mosher RB, Moore JB (1998) The relationship of self-concept and self-care in children with cancer. *Nursing Science Quarterly* **11**(3): 116–22

Nelson-McDermott MA (1993) Learned helplessness as an interacting variable with self-care agency: Testing a theoretical model. *Nursing Science Quarterly* **6**(1): 28–38

Nightingale F (1859) *Notes on Nursing: What It Is and What It Is Not*. Harrison and Sons, London

Nightingale EO, Wolverton L (1993) Adolescent rolelessness in modern society. *Teachers' College* **94**: 472–86

Nolan M, Grant G, Keady J (1996) *Understanding Family Care*. Open University Press, Oxford

Orem D (1971) *Nursing: Concepts of Practice*. CV Mosby, St Louis

Orem D (1980) *Nursing: Concepts of Practice* (2nd Edn). CV Mosby, St Louis

Orem D (1995) *Nursing: Concepts of Practice* (5th Edn). CV Mosby, St Louis

Pearson A, Vaughan B (1986) *Nursing Models for Practice*. Heinemann, Oxford

Pickens JM (1999) Living with serious metnal illness: The desire for normalcy. *Nursing Science Quarterly* **12**(3): 233–9

Popper K (1963) *Conjectures and Refutations: The Growth of Scientific Knowledge*. Harper Row, New York

Riehl JP, Roy C (1980) *Conceptual Models for Nursing Practice*. Appleton-

Century-Crofts, New York

Rogers C (1961) *On Becoming a Person: A Therapist's View of Psychotherapy.* Constable, London

Rolland JS (1994) *Families, Illness and Disability: An Integrative Treatment Model.* Basic Books, New York

Royal College of Nursing (2009) Defining Nursing. http://www.rcn.org.uk/__data/assets/pdf_file/0003/78564/001983.pdf [Accessed 7th July 2009]

Schneider JK, Hornberger S, Booker J, Davis A, Kralich R (1993) A medication discharge planning program. *Clinical Nursing Research* **2**(1): 41–53

Seligman M (1975) *Helplessness: On Depression, Developments and Death.* Freeman, San Francisco

Soderhamn O, Cliffordson C (2001) The structure of self-care in a group of elderly people. *Nursing Science Quarterly* **14**(1): 55–8

Taylor SG (1988) Nursing theory and the nursing process: Orem's theory in practice. *Nursing Science Quarterly* 111–9

Taylor SG (1991) The structure of nursing diagnosis from Orem's theory. *Nursing Science Quarterly* **4**(1): 24–32

Timmins F, Horan P (2001) A critical analysis of the potential contribution of Orem's (2001) self-care deficit nursing theory to contemporary coronary care nursing practice. *European Journal of Cardiovascular Nursing* **6**(1): 32–9

Walker LO, Grobe SJ (1999) The construct of thriving in pregnancy and post-partum. *Nursing Science Quarterly* **12**(2): 151–7

Wilson FL, Mood DW, Risk J, Kershaw T (2003) Evaluation of educational materials using Orem's self-care deficit theory. *Nursing Science Quarterly* **16**(1): 68–76

Zrinyi M, Zekanya RI (2001) Does self-care agency change between hospital admission and discharge? An Orem-based investigation. *International Nursing Review* **54** (3): 256–62

CHAPTER 9

The Roper-Logan-Tierney Model

Introduction

The Roper-Logan-Tierney model of nursing was named after its authors: Nancy Roper, Winifred Logan and Alison Tierney. All three are graduates of the Department of Nursing at the University of Edinburgh and together they have created one of the few nursing models developed outside of North America.

Roper (1976) originally sought to identify a 'core' of nursing which would explicate the 'unity' of nursing. Further identification of the particular knowledge and skills necessary for nursing practice specialties would then explicate its 'diversity'. What she found in her investigation was that the 'core' related to everday living activities and this supported her idea to base a nursing model on a model of living. Logan, a seasoned nursing educator and internationally experienced clinical nurse brought from her travels back to the UK both a keen understanding of the importance of the psychological, sociocultural and environmental factors affecting patients and an education which had included study at Columbia University in New York and exposure to the work of nursing theorists including Virginia Henderson. Tierney joined Roper and Logan as she was restructuring the coursework for a nursing degree programme. She saw the value in organising disparate subjects within the overall framework of a nursing model. The authors have asserted that the model is deliberately uncomplicated and intended to 'assist learners to develop a way of thinking about nursing in general terms'. Tierney's later and ongoing contributions to the development of the model include her years of experience as a nurse researcher (Roper et al., 2000: v-vi).

The authors first published their work in 1980 and, in subsequent publications, they have refined the model to reflect both an evolving academic climate and the changing needs of society. The most recent publication by the authors was compiled as a monograph in 2000. In 2008, Holland et al. published *Applying the Roper Logan Tierney Model in Practice* with the stated purpose of enabling students and teachers to explore the different dimensions of the model through case studies and exercises. At least one author (Fraser, 1996) suggested that the model was declining in popularity. However, there do continue to be publications based on the model and it remains quite popular in the UK, particularly in the public sector and medical-surgical settings. While the 2000 monograph is the last that will be published by the original three authors, they have invited others to continue their work in testing the concepts and refining the model (Roper et al., 2000: x-xi).

The model of living which is the underpinning of the Roper-Logan-Tierney model of nursing aims to simply, yet meaningfully, capture the main features of the complex phenomenon of 'living' (Roper et al., 2000: 13). There are five main components, or concepts: activities of living (ALs), lifespan, dependence/independence continuum, factors influencing ALs, and individuality in living.

The authors describe 12 activities of living in detail: maintaining a safe environment, communicating, breathing, eating and drinking, eliminating, personal cleansing and dressing, controlling body temperature, mobilising, working and playing, expressing sexuality, sleeping, and dying. The four concepts: lifespan, the dependence/independence continuum, ALs and factors influencing ALs are interpreted in terms of their relationships to the 12 ALs, and the synthesis of these interpretations establishes the fifth concept of individuality of living.

The lifespan is the continuum from birth to death. Roper et al. (2000) have identified five stages of life: infancy, childhood, adolescence, adulthood, and senior citizenship. At different stages along the continuum, there are varying degrees of dependence and independence in the activities of living. Also, as individuals move through their lifespan, every aspect of life is influenced by the factors affecting activities of living. These factors, according to Roper et al. (2000), are biological, psychological, sociocultural, environmental, and politico-economic. In terms of the model, individuality can be seen as a product of the influence on the ALs of all the other concepts and the complex interactions among them (Roper et al, 2000: 59–76).

The Roper-Logan-Tierney model of nursing is built upon this model of living and the concepts are very much the same. The one exception is that individuality of living becomes individualising nursing for the practitioner. The assumptions of the model are presented in *Box 9.1* (Roper et al., 2000: 77–143).

In their monograph, Roper et al. analyse and summarise the critiques of their model (2000: 158–65). The criticism in the UK has focused on the oversimplicity, rather than the complexity, of the model; lack of 'fresh' conceptualisation; lack of new perspective on nursing activities; and 'non-challenging', entrenched viewpoints. It is just possible to assume that this critique is based on the comparison of the Roper-Logan-Tierney model, rightly or wrongly, to other nursing theories. However, it is important to keep in mind that the initial starting points for the development of this model

---

Box 9.1. Assumptions of the Roper-Logan-Tierney Model

- Living can be described as an amalgam of activities of living (ALs)
- The way ALs are carried out by each person contributes to individuality in living
- The individual is valued at all stages of the lifespan
- Throughout the lifespan until adulthood, the majority of individuals tend to become increasingly independent in the ALs
- While independence in the ALs is valued, dependence should not diminish the dignity of the individual
- An individual's knowledge about, attitudes to, and behaviour related to ALs are influenced by a variety of factors that can be categorised broadly as biological, psychological, sociocultural, environmental, and politico-economic factors
- The way in which an individual carries out ALs can fluctuate within a range of normal for that person
- When the individual is 'ill', there may be problems (actual or potential) with the ALs
- During the lifespan, most individuals experience significant life events or untoward events which can affect the way they carry out ALs, and may lead to problems, actual or potential
- The concept of potential problems incorporates the promotion and maintenance of health, and the prevention of disease; and identifies the role of the nurse as a health teacher, even in illness settings
- Within a healthcare context, nurses and patients/clients enter into a professional relationship whereby, whenever possible, the patient/client continues to be an autonomous decision-making individual
- Nurses are part of a multiprofessional healthcare team who work in partnership for the benefit of the client/patient, and for the health of the community
- The specific function of nursing is to assist the individual to prevent, alleviate or solve, or cope positively with, problems (actual or potential) related to ALs

(Roper et al., 2001: 79–80)

---

have been quite different and thus it is possible to criticise the critique and its relevance.

Roper et al. (2000: 159) also provide nurses' views and critique from a pragmatic perspective. This brings up issues regarding the conceptual clarity in the form of such questions as: Which AL does bleeding or pain fit into? Also, from clinicians/nurses' perspective, the model seems too problem and hospital oriented. The most relevant criticism seems to be the amount of time it takes to complete the assessment, document it and communicate it. Follow up through to full successful utilisation of the model is similarly challenging. Roper et al. (1983) recognised these challenges as early as 1983 and they suggested working towards shared interprofessional documentation.

A notable point to consider when reviewing the Roper-Logan-Tierney model is that the authors have not developed their model to align with the conceptualisation of nursing metaparadigms. They have, in fact, cited Melies and Trangenstein (1994) who questioned the utility of the metaparadigms to the discipline of nursing. Nonetheless, this chapter provides a discussion of the concepts for consistency and for comparative study.

Nursing

The Roper-Logan-Tierney model for nursing was to some extent influenced by Virginia Henderson's concept of nursing (Roper et al., 1985: 14–15). The authors have quoted Henderson's definition:

> *Nursing is primarily assisting the individual (sick or well) in the performance of those activities contributing to health, or its recovery (or to a peaceful death) that he [patient] would perform unaided if he had the necessary strength, will or knowledge. It is likewise the unique contribution of nursing to help the individual to be independent of such assistance as soon as possible.*
>
> (Roper et al., 1985: 13–14)

The authors further suggest that the nature of nursing and nursing activities may be simple, but that the application to the particular demands of a patient, and the thinking, decision making and action elements make nursing complex, requiring management expertise to co-ordinate all the elements.

The goals of nursing relate to the activities of living. Nursing aims at:

- The individual acquiring, maintaining, or restoring maximum independence in the activities of living, or enabling him or her to cope with dependence on others if circumstances make it necessary.
- Enabling the individual to carry out preventative activities independently to avoid ill health.
- Providing comforting strategies to promote recovery and eventual independence.
- Providing medically described treatments to overcome illness or its symptoms, leading to recovery and eventual independence (see for example, Roper et al., 1980).

Roper et al. (1980, 1985, 2000) have presented a diagrammatic representation of a 'model of nursing' based on the model of living. This visual presentation shows the focus of nursing practice (and nurses' need for knowledge) concerning the biological, physiological, socio-cultural, environmental and politico-economic aspects of the 12 activities of living and the dependence/independence continuum. The diagrammatic representation has undergone alterations since its original version in 1980. The authors explain the alterations in their monograph (Roper et al., 2000: 171–9).

The model outlines identification of problem(s) and the problem solving process, whether these are actual or potential. Roper et al. (2000) states that the role of nursing/nurses is to enable the patient/client to prevent, alleviate/solve, or cope positively with problems (actual or potential) related to ALs and to promote independence in the activities of living (Roper, 1985: 76; Roper et al., 2000: 135–7). The authors describe that the patient's priority may not be the same as the nurse's, and that there may be problems of which the patient is not aware (i.e. nurse-perceived problems), but also that there may be 'a patient-perceived problem' (e.g. particular worry) of which the nurse is not immediately aware. The problem(s) could be a life-threatening emergency or non-emergency, and thus the problems can be prioritised. The patient's priority and nurse's priority regarding the problem may or may not be the same, but the authors assume that when the priorities are the same, this contributes to the motivation to co-operate in carrying out the interventions to achieve the set goals (Roper et al., 1985: 76; 2000: 135–6).

Individualising nursing and nursing process

An important component of the model is the nursing process which, for the authors, is individualised to each patient and engages patients' participation in their own care. The nursing process is interactive and, although described as being comprised of four phases, is also dynamic with continuous feedback. The four phases, assessing, planning, implementing, and evaluating, are therefore not intended to compartmentalise thinking. Instead, each of the four phases is dependent on the effectiveness of the others in a cyclical process (Roper et al., 1985: 14–15; 2000: 122–44).

The assessment is comprised of collecting biographical and health data, comparing current activities of living to the patient's usual routine, identifying the individual's problems with ALs, and identifying priorities among problems. The assessment of the ALs is central to the model of nursing and each of the person's relevant ALs is assessed in the context of the other concepts of the model – life span, dependence/independence,

Table 9.1. Assessing the activities of living	
Assessing the ALs	*Examples of assessment*
Assessing the ability to maintain safe environment	• The nurse needs to assess/know whether or not the person appreciates the dangers in the environment and knows how to prevent accidents
Assessing communication skills	• The nurse needs to asses/observe whether the person is reticent or forthcoming when talking about home and health problems
Assessing breathing	• Physiological assessment • The nurse should attempt to discover also the person's perceptions of multiple ill-effects of smoking and whether or not help with giving up or reducing the habit of smoking would be welcomed
Assessing eating and drinking habits	• When nursing under or overweight patients, the nurse needs to talk/assess what, when and how much the person eats/drinks (alcohol consumption)
Assessing the elimination habits	• The assessment associated with bowel and urinary function/dysfunction is always sensitive
Assessing personal cleansing habits and dressing	• The nurse assesses brushing the teeth, hand-washing, skin status (bruising) and risk of developing pressure ulcers
Assessing control of body temperature	• Temperature. The nurse may also assess flushing of the skin, excessive respiration, presence of goose flesh, shivering and cold/hot hands/feet
Assessing mobility	• The nurse assesses stiffness of the joints and posture
Assessing work and play routines	• The nurse gains understanding through the assessment what the person considers challenging and what is boring or stressful; employment/unemployment
Assessing the ALs of expressing sexuality	• The nurse gains understanding how people express their gender – mode of dress, use of cosmetics • The assessment is always sensitive; may based on cues which are expressions of sexuality
Assessing sleeping routines	• The nurse assesses routines and use of medications
Assessing the needs of the dying	• Becomes essential only when the diagnosis and prognosis indicate that the person's death is probable • Assessment requires sensitivity and observation whether or not the person wants to talk about the many aspects associated with death and dying
	(Roper et al., 2001: 130–4)

the five factors influencing ALs, and, therefore, the patient's individuality in living (Roper et al., 1985: 72–6; 2000: 124–36). Examples of the assessments of the activities of living are presented in the *Table 9.1*.

Assessing is not a one time only activity, rather additional data are collected as the nurse has further opportunities to observe and talk/listen to the person in the course of her work. The amount and type of information collected about the ALs varies and, depending on circumstances, all of the information on all the ALs may not always be relevant. Therefore, assessing is not a rigid routine, carried out at a particular time and in a particular way, but it is an ongoing activity and one that requires tailoring to the circumstances of the individual person. Assessing is applicable to people who are in the healthcare system for surveillance, investigation or treatment of illness. Identification of problem(s) is also applicable when it comes to health maintenance and promotion, because the aim is to identify and avoid potential problems with the ALs as well (Roper et al., 1985: 72–6; 2000: 130–5). During the assessment the nurse needs to take into account the stage of the lifespan and to consider the person's 'previous routines' and how these may have been fashioned by biological, socio-cultural, environmental, politico-economic factors and what the person can/cannot do independently (Roper et al., 2000: 130–5).

Planning is comprised of setting goals and preparing a nursing plan. The objective of the planning is to (1) prevent identified potential problems with any of the ALs from becoming actual, (2) to solve identified actual problems, (3) where possible, to alleviate the problems that cannot be solved, (4) to help the person cope positively with those problems that cannot be alleviated, (5) to prevent recurrence of a treated problem, and (6) to help the person to be as comfortable and pain-free as possible when death is inevitable (Roper et al., 2000: 137; see also Roper et al., 1985: 76). The goals (short- and long-term) are set to each actual and potential problem and these are stated in terms of outcomes that are possible to observe, measure or test, so that their subsequent evaluation is likely to be accomplished (and documented with time and date). The nursing plan, that is based on the model, tells what to do and when. It contains the stated goals or desired outcomes for each problem, a date by which the goal(s) are expected to be achieved and the nursing interventions (and patient participation) to achieve the goals (Roper et al., 1986: 77; 2000: 137–40).

The activities associated with the implementation of the plan include both planned activities and those that may be unplanned. The evaluation is the comparison of what has been achieved to the objective/set goals. This is an important component and the documentation that the authors suggest is critical to establishing how nursing processes benefit patients (Roper et al., 1985: 14; 2000: 140–3).

Health

There is an interesting article (Roper et al., 1983) in which the authors discuss the problem-orientated approach that works well within their model for nursing. For the authors, it would seem that health is conceptualised as the ability to function independently in relation to the 12 ALs (Fitzpatrick and Whall, 1989). They believe that the focus on problems has not narrowed their concept of nursing to problem-solving only. They state,

> *If anything, we now understand better the nurse's role in prevention of ill-health and promotion of health using a problem-oriented approach to the nursing process.*
>
> (Roper et al., 1983)

In the 2000 monograph, Roper et al. categorically reject health promotion as incompatible with paradigms such as their model. In fact, they state

> *We believe that our model is entirely congruent with the ever-increasing emphasis on healthy lifestyle and healthy public policy.*
>
> (Roper et al., 2000: 156)

Roper et al. discuss the concept of health from a very broad perspective (2000: 109–14). The authors acknowledge that from the socio-cultural perspective health status has an effect on role(s), and state that culture influences the way societies deal with health and illness. The important point that is made regarding the 'concept of health' is that an individual's health behaviour and varied responses to illness are strongly impacted by socio-cultural factors, and understanding these requires knowledge of social, cultural, spiritual, religious and ethical issues (see also Roper et al., 1985: 24–6, 54–62).

Health and its relation to politico-economic factors are illuminated from political, economic and legal perspectives. The authors acknowledge that health is firmly rooted in prevailing political, economic and social realities and that health is not only impacted by the healthcare services, but all fields of public policy, legal activities, industrialisation and economy (Roy et al., 2000: 118–22, see also Roper et al., 1985: 24–6, 54–62).

Person

The model conceptualises the person as a biological being with inseparable mind and body. The model represents the individual, the subject of nursing, engaged in the process of living. Roper (1976) described the person (i.e. subject of nursing) as follows:

> *Basically, man is envisaged as carrying out various activities during a lifespan from conception to death. His/her main objective is to attain self-fulfilment and maximum independence in each activity of daily living within the limitations set by his particular circumstances. He/she also carries out many activities of preventing, comforting and seeking nature and he appropriately alter priorities among the activities of daily living. In these ways, the individual endeavours to be healthy and independent in the process of living.*

Each individual/person has a lifespan from birth to death, but its length is variable. The individual's/person's stages of the life span have been described as follows: (pre-natal stage/conception*) infancy (0–5 years*), childhood (6–12 years*), adolescence (13–18 years*), adulthood (18–65 years*) and old age (65+*) (Roper et al., 1985: 66–69*, 2000: 86–94). The lifespan and its different stages are closely related to the ALs/nursing and the concept of dependence and independence (Roper et al., 1985: 69–71; 2000: 95–114).

The concept of dependence/independence is described in the context of the 12 ALs. The levels of dependence/independence are depicted as a continuum. In the diagrammatic presentation of the model this is illustrated as an arrow that indicates that movement can be in either direction. This concept is interesting, since it is related to circumstances and its interpretation is based on a nurse's judgement. In general, a person is encouraged to achieve or regain maximum independence. However, there are circumstances (e.g. unconsciousness) when individuals are totally dependent on nurses and this may not even be their desire (e.g. immobilisation in traction). Therefore, the concept of dependence/independence is evolving: sometimes a person is helped towards independence in the ALs and at other times a person is helped to accept the dependence (Roper et al., 1985: 69–71; 2000: 98–9).

The conceptual presentation of the person includes a description of biological (anatomical and physiological) terms. A person's body, its biological state, is constantly changing and this is partly determined by the individual's genetic inheritance. The conceptual presentation of a person includes also the description of psychological terms (intellectual and emotional aspects) and these are seen to be related to the biological, socio-cultural, environmental and politico-economic factors as well (Roper et al., 2000: 60–4, 105–8; see also Roper et al., 1985: 28–53).

Environment

Roper et al. (1985: 83–107; 2000: 114–18), while not presenting the environment as a metaparadigm, have nonetheless discussed it in the context of maintaining a safe environment and also as a factor influencing ALs. In many ways, they have been quite literal in noting humankind's progress in controlling the external environment such that most no longer live under the constant threat of natural forces. They illustrate, however, that some threats remain, such as earthquakes, floods and fires, and they also highlight threats such as radiation, chemical waste, modern war weaponry and the illicit use of drugs which have been created by humankind itself.

In the model of living, the authors present environmental factors such as light and sound waves, organic and inorganic particles, the natural habitat, and the built environment. Among the potential hazards in the environment, they include external agents that can cause injury, stress that impacts biological, psychological and socio-cultural aspects of a person, and abuse that can cause physical or mental harm. As far as hospitals are concerned as an environment, the authors point out the inevitable risk of exposure to different types of pathogens, the importance of preventing their spread, and concern about the increasing incidences of hospital acquired (drug resistant) infections. They acknowledge that the examples they discuss are merely representative of the components that comprise the environment. Generally, they state that the nurse should consider all environmental factors that can impact or potentially impact a patient in either a negative or positive way (Roper et al., 2000: 16–18, 114–18).

Clinical application: Orthopaedic nursing

Deborah Smith is a 45-year-old waitress who works in a local fine dining restaurant. She lives with her husband Peter (50 years old) who is the executive chef in the same restaurant. The couple have no children, but they have two dogs. They have been living in the same house in the centre of a small town for 20 years. One evening when Mrs Smith was walking home from work the road was icy and her shoes were slippery. She fell to the ground with her hand/palm outstretched. Mrs Smith was taken to the emergency department by a neighbour who was at the scene when the accident happened. An x-ray confirmed a left radius fracture. A distal radius fracture (Colle's fracture) is a common fracture and because of its proximity to the wrist joint, it is often called a wrist fracture. Treatment is usually with immobilisation, although surgery is sometimes needed for complex fractures (Black et al., 2001: 617–19; Lemone and Burke, 2004: 1205).

When Mrs Smith arrived at the emergency department, she was quite upset about the accident. Her wrist was swollen and tender, but the skin was intact. The colour of the fingers/skin was pink/normal and the radial pulse was palpable. There was some numbness in the hand, but there was no loss of sensation in the fingers. Mrs Smith reported that she could see a 'bump' and deformity on the wrist and that she could not move her hand. There were no other injuries due to the fall on the forearm, elbow or shoulder. She also expressed concern about her work, getting home to her dogs and being able to keep up her household chores. Mrs Smith had a cast put on her wrist/hand and was discharged home within a few hours.

The patient problems relating to the activities of living are identified during assessment and transferred to the plan of care. The goals, agreed upon by the patient and the nurse, using the Roper-Logan-Tierney model, are centred around the patient achieving independence in the activities of living or coping with any dependencies he/she may have. The overriding goal is for the patient to agree to the way in which goals are achieved and the schedule for achieving them as fully as possible. The Roper-Logan-Tierney model focuses on the behaviour of the individual, and this needs to be reflected in the problem and goal statements in the care plan. This approach is seen as essential to the evaluation of the appropriateness and effectiveness of the nursing intervention. The actual and potential problems for Mrs Smith are shown in *Table 9.2*.

In this example, the goals (i.e. outcomes which will indicate independence or coping with dependence) would read that Mrs Smith: (1) will maintain her independence regarding (a) personal cleaning and dressing and (b) elimination during the time she is wearing the cast; (2) will be able to continue preparing the meals at home; (3) the flexibility of the fingers and muscle strength of her left hand will remain at the same level or rise; (4) will be able to get rest/sleep without pain during the nights. Since Mrs Smith is an adult and she has no history of health problems, the nursing aims will be to prevent any potential problems that may in any way affect her health status and independence.

The nursing actions that the nurse and Mrs Smith are taking to overcome the problems, prevent the potential problems and achieve the goals are mainly educational with the provision of information. Mrs Smith's environment at home was considered safe and she herself had recognised the probable safety hazards. The nurse discusses with Mrs Smith the possibility of using a harness for the dogs or walking them one at a time. She also advises her to use firm shoes when going out with the dogs in order to avoid falls or accidents. The nurse discusses with Mrs Smith about the pain and swelling of the fingers, listens carefully and explains the use of the pain medications that the physician has prescribed. The nurse also provides information regarding other ways to relieve the pain and swelling/oedema, such as the use of pillows to elevate the hand/cast and ice-bags during the day aand at night. The nurse provides written information regarding mobilisation/exercises for the hand/fingers and exercises to increase muscle strength. She coordinates a consultation with a physiotherapist for further assessment. She also appraises Mrs Smith of the timeline for having her wrist and cast checked by her family physician who will evaluate how well her recovery is progressing.

Table 9.2 Assessing the activities of living

Activity	Usual routine	Actual/potential problem
Maintaining a safe environment	• Mrs Smith has a very busy lifestyle. She does all the work at home: cooking, grocery shopping, cleaning, laundry and gardening • She takes care of the grooming, feeding and walking/running of the two dogs. The dogs are large and not well behaved; she needs both hands to manage their leashes	Environment: • Mrs Smith recognises the hazards to her safety at home. She could easily drop large or heavy objects when trying to manage with only one hand • Recognises the hazards to her safety of going out with the dogs. She coud lose her balance and fall if the dogs pull her
Communication	• Mrs Smith is alert and oriented. She remembered everything that had happened: how she fell and that she had not hit her head during the fall. She communicated fluently and coherently	Psychological: • Mrs Smith does not seem particularly anxious, but regards it as a nuisance which might interfere with her usual activities for some time • She experiences/expresses pain
Breathing	• Mrs Smith has never smoked, but she has been exposed to tobacco smoke regularly at the restaurant.	Environment: • Mrs Smith has no current/history of respiratory problems, but may be more sensitive to respiratory problems/infections
Eating and drinking	• Mrs Smith enjoys cooking at home; she has a good appetite, has never had indigestion and has never been overweight. She also pays attention to 'healthy' eating	Physical: • Mrs Smith may need some minimal help (e.g. shopping, cutting food, carrying a tray) at home because she cannot use her left hand due to immobilisation with the cast.
Eliminating	• Mrs Smith is passing urine normally and the bowel pattern is regular, usually daily	Physical: • Mrs Smith may have difficulties with hygiene after elimination due to the immobilisation of her left hand • Mrs Smith needs minimal or occasional help in the bathroom/toilet, because she cannot use her left hand

Activity of living	Assessment	Problems
Personal cleaning and dressing	● Mrs Smith takes a shower every morning; she blow dries her hair and applies make-up ● She appears clean and well cared for	Physical: ● Cannot get full shower(s) with the cast on the left hand. Mrs Smith may manage all personal care with minimal help (i.e. assistance in the shower/washing, using the towel, and help with clothing) ● Her fingers are swollen and the wedding ring(s) and the wrist watch needs to be taken off immediately
Controlling body temperature	● Mrs Smith's temperature on admission was 36.4°C.	Physical: ● Mrs. Smith's has a jacket, but the sleeve does not fit over the cast. She can cope with changes in environmental temperatures at discharge ● Mrs Smith has to wear clothes that have sleeve(s) wide enough to go over the cast
Mobilising	● Mrs Smith calls herself an 'out-door' person. She exercises regularly, walks and runs with her dogs	● There are no actual or potential problems inhibiting Mrs Smith's optimum mobility ● Potential problem: stiffness of fingers due to the immobilisation for which she needs to exercise the fingers six times daily
Working and playing	● Mrs Smith works as a waitress in a local restaurant. During the day/night, she serves lunch/dinner dishes and carries heavy trays	Physical: ● Mrs Smith may not be able carry heavy dishes or trays if her muscle strength deteriorates during the immobilisation
Expressing sexuality	● Mrs Smith is very comfortable expressing her sexuality and talking about her sex life with her husband	Physical: ● Mrs Smith expresses concern about the cast affecting the couple's sex life
Sleeping	● Mrs Smith sleeps well at night and she shares the bed with her husband. She likes to sleep on her right or left side. She does not use any sleeping medications	Physical: ● Mrs Smith may not sleep well because of the cast on her left hand. She has to sleep on her back and keep the hand elevated with pillows due to the swelling ● Pain may cause a sleep deficit
Dying	N/A	N/A

Case studies

Thompson (1989) describes in this article the care given to a patient, Tom Mulligan, aged 74, with a chronic leg ulcer. The Roper-Logan-Tierney (1996) model of nursing was used as a basis to assess, plan, implement and evaluate the nursing care given. The author concludes that the model provided a holistic framework for the assessment of the patient's needs. This case study is very interesting because it also provides a comparison of costs and cost-effectiveness for two different types of leg ulcer treatments.

Rowe (1995) reports in this paper on nursing a person who had suffered a myocardial infarction (MI). The life-threatening experience of an acute MI stimulates a wide variety of physical and psychological responses for both the person and his family. The nurse's role in assisting a person through a major life crisis from a dependent to an independent status is described. The Roper-Logan-Tierney model for nursing seems to provide a suitable framework for nursing a person who has suffered an MI. The framework to care ensures that maximum health potential is achieved.

O'Connor and Timmins (2002) decribe the use of the Roper-Logan-Tierney model in a neonatal intensive care unit. This paper examines nurses' views on the model as described in the literature. It also examines the model's usefulness in a neonatal care unit and focuses on the care of a premature baby, using the model as a basis for assessment and care.

Healy and Timmins (2003) explore in this paper the use of the Roper-Logan-Tierney nursing model in a neonatal transport setting. The article provides an overview of the model and describes the background information on a selected patient, followed by a detailed assessment of this patient using the activities of living. The article provides also an evaluation of the use of the model in this clinical situation with reference to literature on the topic.

Timmins and O'Shea (2004) report in this article the use of the Roper-Logan-Tierney model in assessing, planning, implementing and evaluating the care of an infant in a neonatal intensive care setting. The paper also provides an insight into a student's reflection upon learning during the programme and preparation of a care study. The Roper-Logan-Tierney model seems to provide a clear framework to guide the nursing care of the neonate. Individualisation of nursing practice was a particular benefit that emerged during this study. Rather than focusing on the medical and routine day-to-day aspects of care in the neonatal unit, the use of the model allowed for the construction of a plan of care based on the baby's own specific physical, social and emotional needs.

Mooney and O'Brien (2006) report a case study, using the Roper-Logan-Tierney model of nursing. The authors examine the presentation of a patient with a history of drug misuse and a current diagnosis of infective endocarditis and hepatitis C. While the model of nursing incorporates 12 activities of daily living, this case study deals with three specific activities: maintaining a safe environment, communication and breathing. One of the main concerns arising from this study was the inadequate management of pain for the patient. This finding is interesting, since the earlier critique of the study has questioned the model's sensitivity in the assessment of pain.

Empirical studies

Mason (1999) reports a project that investigated how nursing care plans were being used in five clinical areas, and assessed their influence on nursing practice. An exploratory, predominantly qualitative research design was selected utilising participant observation (110 hours), tape-recorded focus group interviews, and diaries (one week). In four of the five clinical areas, the 'activities of daily living' section of the care plans had no apparent positive influence on nursing practice which was driven by other factors and sources of information. Care plans in the remaining ward were clinically led and locally owned, and they operated as an important guide to practice. The author concludes that a reinvention of the nursing care plan is needed without the constraint of a nursing model as its necessary foundation. The author further recommends that new and imaginative plans of action for patient care should be encouraged, developed at ward level, and tailored to the demands of the clinical area. These should contain a minimum of documentation and integration with nursing practice. The study is very interesting, but the findings are limited due to the purposive selection of the wards.

Murphy et al. (2000) report an empirical study that was aimed at determining whether the Roper-Logan-Tierney model was an appropriate model for planning nursing care for clients who are mentally ill. Data were collected from two sources. A care plan audit was used to evaluate the extent to which the model was used to assess, plan and evaluate nursing care in nursing documentation. The audit tool was comprised of 22 questions, divided into three sections. A total of 237 care plans was collected. Qualitative interviews with 20 nurses explored their experiences of using the model and their perceptions of the model's usefulness and appropriateness for planning care. Both data sets were complementary: the qualitative data providing contextual information which helped put the findings into perspective. It was found that there was little evidence that the Roper-Logan-Tierney model guided care planning and that goals and nursing interventions were frequently not explicitly documented. Interviews with nurses indicated that they lacked educational preparation for using the model and found the model constraining and physically orientated. The authors of this paper conclude that the appropriateness of the model for planning care for clients who are mentally ill is questioned. The authors' recommendation is that nurses need to be adequately prepared if they are to use a model appropriately. An important observation is that consideration should be given when selecting a model as to its 'fit' with the needs of the client group and the ward team philosophy.

Kara (2007) conducted a study to determine whether the Roper-Logan-Tierney model of nursing care affects the outcomes of patients with chronic obstructive pulmonary disease (COPD). The study design was an experimental style. The sample consisted of 60 subjects with a diagnosis of COPD who were hospitalised in a university hospital (Erzurum, Turkey) in 2001. The subjects were randomly selected into control and experimental groups. On admission, the researcher completed a nursing diagnosis form for COPD for each patient, consisting of demographic characteristics and an assessment nursing diagnosis for each of the patients. Control group patients were treated by routine nursing care while the experimental group patients were treated by nursing care according to the Roper-Logan-Tierney model. Upon discharge, nursing diagnoses were assessed again in both control and experimental groups. Although there was no statistically significant decrease in most nursing diagnoses in the control group, there was a significant decrease in nursing diagnoses in favour of the experimental group. The study demonstrated that there were improvements in patient outcomes in the concept of holistic and individualised nursing care of patients with COPD according to the Roper-Logan-Tierney model. The author concludes that the findings of this study have practical importance for nursing practice. Using the Roper-Logan-Tierney model in the care of patients with COPD seems to serve as an efficient guide for nurses, patients and family members to participate and facilitate the effectiveness of patient care.

Practice development studies

Bellman (1996) reports a project that was undertaken in two phases over a 15-month period utilising an action research approach. In phase one, triangulation of the data enabled the 12 practitioners/co-researchers to identify and reflect on patients' psychological needs within the independence/dependence continuum of the Roper et al. (1990) model on a 22-bed surgical ward. Phase two involved a collaborative approach to the planning, implementation and evaluation of innovations that resulted from reflection on practice. The most significant congruent perception, elicited from triangulation of the patient and practitioner data sources during phase one, revealed the need to address the psychological factors. The practitioners believed that they needed to develop this concept further in practice. A psychologically safe environment was developed in phase two. Group reflection was seen as an essential feedback strategy during the change process. This study demonstrated in a very interesting way the practitioners' varying levels of knowledge, conceptualisation of the model in practice, and why many experienced difficulties relating the theory to practice.

Webb and Pontin (1997) discuss in this paper a care plan audit that was carried out as part of an action research project involving the introduction of primary nursing. The audit was composed of six sections. The first five referred to the strategies involved in identifying and responding to patient's problems and the last focused on evaluating the degree to which all documentation was completed comprehensively. The tool's section dealing with patient assessment was based on the Roper-Logan-Tierney activities of living model and the nursing process. The audit showed that few changes in documentation had taken place as a result of the introduction of primary nursing and that the volume of communications had increased. However, much of this was not documented on care plans. The study confirmed that the challenge was how to educate nurses to document nursing assessments and care planning. This paper is an interesting example of the utilisation of the model as a framework for an audit tool.

McLafferty and Farley (2007) report in this paper on the nursing management of delirium. Delirium is a common and under-reported problem in older adults and it can have a negative effect on patient outcomes. Nurses often fail to identify it. This article outlines nursing interventions based on the Roper-Logan-Tierney model of the activities of living. The authors use the model to highlight the risk factors of delirium and thus demonstrate the use of the model as an initial assessment framework. The article outlines nursing measures that can be implemented by staff to reduce and minimise the effects of delirium.

Suggested further reading

- Keen and Malby (1992) discuss organisational changes in the UK. The study shows that the six organisations that were the research sites were inflexible in their design and would not allow the incorporation of different nursing models and practices. All the sites were heavily dependent on the Roper-Logan-Tierney (1980) model of nursing.
- Richardson and Poole (2001) focus discussion in this paper on chronic pain, coping and the proposed role for nurses and nursing models. Activity of living based nurse models such as that proposed by Roper, Logan and Tierney are utilised commonly to rationalise, structure and guide practice. The authors propose that when using a model in the context of chronic pain, this should be extended to incorporate the assessment of coping and its effect on disability.

It is argued in this paper that the need for reliable and valid means to assess coping are of paramount importance as this will facilitate and inform the treatment and management of chronic pain. A classification system which categorises chronic pain patients in terms of how they function in daily life as either adaptive copers, interpersonally distressed or dysfunctional is outlined. The similarities between this and a routine nursing assessment based on the activities of living model are highlighted. The authors propose that the innovative use of nursing activity of living models could provide the framework for a pain clinic based assessment of coping that has greater utility for professionals and patients alike.

- Timmons (2003) talks about nurses' resistance to the implementation and use of computer systems. The problems with the way the Roper-Logan-Tierney model and the nursing process are implemented within the system are addressed in this paper. The key argument is that the dependence/independence continuum and the lifespan are important factors in the Roper-Logan-Tierney model. However, none of the systems in use explicitly included these factors. The problem is then that when excluding these parts and concentrating on the 12 activities of daily living, the care given can become reductionistic and mechanical.

- Hyde et al. (2006) present in this paper an analysis of nursing records in order to understand the structural and social processes that mediate the texts. Forty-five sets of nursing records drawn from four clinical sites were subjected to a discourse analysis. This article focuses on discussing two main findings: (1) the manner in which nurses controlled, regulated and invigilated patients' activities of daily living and (2) the way in which activities of daily living were mediated by a biomedical world view in the clinical settings. The authors argue that in the nursing documentation, biochemical interventions in the form of various medications were the most dominant means through which nurses attempted to restore or improve the functional capacity of an activity of daily living. Despite the wide use of the Roper-Logan-Tierney model, the authors conclude that this was little more than a paper exercise with a predominantly medical approach to care by nurses.

References

Bellman LM (1996) Changing nursing practice through reflection on the Roper, Logan and Tierney model: The enhancement approach to action research. *Journal of Advanced Nursing* **24**(1): 129–38

Black J, Hokanson Hawks J, Keene A (2001) *Medical-Surgical Nursing. Clinical Management for Positive Outcomes*. 6th edn. W.B. Saunders Company, Philadelphia, Pennsylvania

Fitzpatrick J, Whall A (1989) *Conceptual Models of Nursing: Analysis and Application*. 2nd edn. London, Prentice Hall Int

Fraser M (1996) *Using Conceptual Models in Practice: Research Based Approach*. 2nd Edn. Harper & Row, London

Healy P, Timmins F (2003) Using the Roper-Logan-Tierney model in neonatal transport. *British Journal of Nursing* 12(13): 792–8

Holland K, Jenkins J, Solomon J, Whittam S (2008) *Applying the Roper-Logan-Tierney Model in Practice*. 2nd edn. Churchill Livingstone, Elsevier

Hyde A, Treacy MM, Scott AP, Mac Neela P, Butler M, Drennan J, Kate I, Byrne A (2006) Social regulation, medicalisation and the nurse's role: Insights from an analysis of nursing documentation. *International Journal of Nursing Studies* 43(6): 735–44

Kara M (2007) Using the Roper, Logan and Tierney Model in care of people with COPD. *Journal of Clinical Nursing* 16(7b): 223–33, July 2007

Keen J, Malby R (1992) Nursing power and practice in the United Kingdom National Health Service. *Journal of Advanced Nursing* 17(7): 863–70

Lemone P, Burke K (2004) *Medical-Surgical Nursing. Critical Thinking in Client Care*. Pearson Prentice Hall, New Jersey

Mason C (1999) Guide to practice or 'load of rubbish'? The influence of care plans on nursing practice in five clinical areas in Northern Ireland. *Journal of Advanced Nursing* 29(2): 380–7

McLafferty E, Farley A (2007) Delirium part two: Nursing management. *Nursing Standard* 21(30): 42–6

Meleis A, Tranguestein P (1994) Facilitating transitions: Redefinition of the nursing mission. *Nursing Outlook* 42: 255–9

Mooney M, O'Brien F (2006) Developing a plan of care using the Roper, Logan and Tierney Model. *British Journal of Nursing* 15(16): 887–92

Murphy K, Cooney A, Casey D, Connor M, O'Connor, Dineen B (2000) The Roper, Logan and Tierney (1996) Model: Perceptions and operationalization of the model in psychiatric nursing within a Health Board in Ireland. *Journal of Advanced Nursing* 31(6): 1333–41

O'Connor M, Timmins F (2002) Using the Roper, Logan and Tierney model in a neonatal ICU. *Professional Nurse* 17(9): 527–30

Richardson C, Poole H (2001) Chronic pain and coping: A proposed role for nurses and nursing models. *Journal of Advanced Nursing* 34(5): 659–67

Roper N (1976) A model for nursing and nursology. *Journal of Advanced Nursing* 1(3): 219–27

Roper N, Logan W, Tierney A (1980) *The Elements of Nursing*. Churchill Livingstone, London

Roper N, Logan W, Tierney A (1983) A Model for Nursing. *Nursing Times* 2: 24–7

Roper N, Logan W, Tierney A (1985) *The Elements of Nursing*. 2nd edn. Churchill Livingstone, Longman Group, Edinburgh

Roper N, Logan W, Tierney A (1986) Nursing models: A process of construction and refinement. In Salvage J, Kershaw B (Eds.) *Models for Nursing*. John Wiley, Chichester. 27–40

Roper N, Logan W, Tierney A (1990) *The Elements of Nursing*. 3rd edn. Churchill Livingstone, London

Roper N, Logan W, Tierney A (2000) *The Roper-Logan-Tierney Model of Nursing: Based on Activities of Living*. Churchill Livingstone, London

Rowe K (1995) Nursing a person who had suffered a myocardial infarction. British *Journal of Nursing* **4**(3): 148–54

Thompson A (1989) Working the system. *Nursing Times* **94**(24): 71–2

Timmins F, O'Shea J (2004) The Roper-Logan-Tierney (1996) model of nursing as a tool for professional development in education. *Nurse Education in Practice* **4**(3): 159–67

Timmons S (2003) Nurses resisting information technology. *Nursing Inquiry* **10**(4): 257–69

Webb C, Pontin D (1997) Evaluating the introduction of primary nursing: The use of a care plan audit. *Journal of Clinical Nursing* **6**(5): 395–401

CHAPTER 10

The Tidal Model of mental health recovery and reclamaton

First developed in England in the late 1990s, the Tidal Model of mental health recovery and reclamation (Barker and Buchanan-Barker, 2005) is recognised internationally as a mid-range nursing theory (Brookes, 2005; in press) but increasingly it is practised by a range of disciplines in the mental health field (Barker and Buchanan-Barker, 2008a). Over 100 Tidal projects, in Australia, Canada, England, Ireland, Japan, New Zealand, Scotland and Wales serve people in youth, acute psychiatric, rehabilitation, autistic-spectrum, learning disability and older persons' services, across the community and hospital care spectrum (see www.tidal-model.com).

The Tidal Model is defined as focusing on helping people who have experienced some metaphorical 'breakdown' recover their lives as fully as possible, by reclaiming the personal story of their distress and difficulty. From hereon we shall use the diminutive, Tidal, popularised by Brookes (2005) to refer to the discrete philosophy which underpins the various approaches embedded within the Tidal Model in practice.

Although applied primarily in the 'mental health' arena, Tidal could be used to address an individual's lived experience of any problem of human living from 'living with a chronic ailment' to 'confronting death'(Barker, 2000a, b).

Although the development of Tidal began only in 1996 (Barker, 1998), it derives from our work with people with 'multiple disabilities' and a diagnosis of 'manic depression' in the early 1980s (Barker and Buchanan-Barker, 2008b). (We use quotes for all diagnostic and other labelling devices to emphasise that we do not, necessarily, agree with the use of such terminology.) Those experiences led us to the realisation that we were working too hard in trying to change people through 'therapy' or some other active form of 'intervention'. Over time we concluded that the most important consideration was not how to change people but to ask: 'How could we help people live a more personally meaningful life by using the personal and interpersonal resources they already possess?' (Barker, 1990).

Our first major influence was Bateson's (1973) proposition that 'a difference which makes a difference is an idea'. It was 'nonsense to say that a man was frightened by a lion, because a lion is not an idea. The man makes an idea of the lion' (Bateson, 1973: 242). In the same context it is nonsense to say, for example, that 'a person has a problem with mental illness'. Rather, if a person is said to have such a problem, it is with the idea that they have such a problem. It has become commonplace to claim that evidence exists for the 'biological basis' of 'mental illness'. We support the view that the 'mind' cannot be 'ill' (other than metaphorically speaking). If biological anomalies are identified, then such states will (automatically) become 'physical illnesses/disorders'. Alzheimer's disease is, clearly, a physical disorder with 'mental' symptoms, but is not a 'mental illness'. To date, we are aware of no unequivocal evidence to recast 'schizophrenia', 'bipolar disorder', 'borderline personality disorder', etc., as 'physical' illnesses.

Later, in the early 1980s, we discovered the work of Shoma Morita who had developed a highly original form of psychotherapy in 1920s Japan. Morita called his 'patients' students, affirming that his role was not to fix or change them (and certainly not to 'rid them' of 'mental illness'), but to help them learn something directly from life, about their experience of living with such problems. In Tidal we have employed Morita's famous maxim 'Do what needs to be done'.

Morita reminded us that, although change is rarely easy, if we are to live more effective and meaningful lives, we must act, not just sit around talking about how we feel about life (Morita et al, 1998). Life cannot be controlled, but we can do something to respond to the challenges life lays before us. This resonates with other, more solution-oriented, contemporary influences on Tidal (Vaughn et al, 1995). However, despite the emphasis on conversation within the Tidal Model, all such discourse (we use 'discourse' here in the commonly-accepted sense, meaning conversation with others, through speech or writing) serves only as a rehearsal for later action within the person's life.

Distinguishing features

The concept of 'recovery' is becoming widely accepted within mental health nursing. However, Tidal possesses some distinctive features. It was

- The first recovery-focused model developed by mental health nurses for mental health nursing practice.
- The first mental health recovery model developed conjointly by mental health professionals and people in their care.
- The first mental health recovery model developed for use in the most challenging situations, i.e. where people are 'at their lowest ebb'.
- The first mental health recovery model to be evaluated rigorously in public sector practice.

- The first model to be used as the basis of recovery-focused care across the hospital–community spectrum – from child and adolescent services to older persons (see Barker and Buchanan-Barker, 2008b; Buchanan-Barker and Barker, 2008).

Philosophy and practice

Although described as both a theory and a model (Brookes, 2005) Tidal is primarily a philosophy for practice: a way of thinking about 'what needs to be done' to enable recovery. Tidal is primarily an approach, or a mind-set, a discrete attitude or disposition, which predetermines how the nurse will interpret and respond to any given situation. Although we have proposed several examples of how this enabling might take place, these serve only as templates for specific individual and group processes (described later). They are illustrative, rather than prescriptive. Practitioners need to tailor each and every interaction, to suit the changing nature of the person's life situation.

Fundamental Tidal propositions

Tidal philosophy embraces discrete theoretical propositions concerning the person-in-care, the nature of the person's problems, how these are represented and what might need to be done to address them. (A range of terms are used in the mental health field: 'patient', 'client', 'user', 'consumer' to refer to those requiring, or receiving care. To acknowledge the 'person-centred' nature of Tidal practice, we advocate use of the term 'person-in-care'.) Here we address the person's problems from the perspective of Fawcett's metaparadigm. Tidal could be framed as a 'paradigm', from Kuhn's perspective (Kuhn, 1970). However, we acknowledge that the field of mental health nursing and mental healthcare (in general) is inherently pre-paradigmatic. Tidal as a paradigm offers an organisational framework, with concepts, theory, assumptions, beliefs, values and principles, which determine how the practitioner will interpret the work of nursing (i.e. enabling the person's recovery). In the 'mental health' field it is, however, only one 'paradigm' among many.

Person

Person as story

Proposition 1: Persons are no more, or less, than story: the stories people tell about their experience of themselves and the wider world of experience, and stories told about them by others.

Despite 50 years of interest in 'person-centred' approaches (Rogers, 1961) professional and policy jargon is still dominated by talk about patients, clients, service users or consumers, and the symptoms, associated with one diagnosis or another. Most professionals (including nurses) betray a need to define those they work with as some kind of 'other'. Despite contemporary references to 'social inclusion', much professional language maintains the practice of 'othering', whereby the 'person-in-care' is excluded from the human pool to which the professional belongs, perhaps as a way of managing the anxiety involved in acknowledging them as 'persons' (Menzies-Lyth, 1959/1988).

For over 25 years we have tried to encourage talk about people who experience some kind of problem in living (Barker, 1982:1). Tidal is concerned with what might be called 'personology', rather than 'pathology' or 'psychology'. In Tidal the stories people tell are alive, ever-changing and beyond reduction. We cannot explain them by reference to biological functions or psychological schemas, any more than we could explain a character in a television soap opera by reference to audio-visual technology; or the message of a Shakespeare play through use of a dictionary or rules of grammar.

Traditionally the fields of psychiatry, psychology and psychotherapy have developed specific narratives about persons, articulating their various 'clinical features', 'symptoms', 'personality traits', etc. Rather than attribute labels to the person, Tidal seeks to learn how people describe their personal experiences, as they relate a story of their personhood.

We accept that who people are and how they become those persons, is influenced by a wide range of physical (biology, etc.) social (families, friends) and cultural (conventions, rituals) factors. However, from the moment of birth (if not during pregnancy) the 'person' is constructed through stories told (or written) by others. At some point, the 'person' will begin to relate her/his own story, generating the story conflict, which often is the source of much interpersonal (if not also political/international) struggle.

Health

Problems in living

Proposition 2: Human life is in a constant state of flow. Incessant change characterises the physical life of the body (which is perpetually regenerating), the person's relations with others and the world in general, and present the person with various problems in living. The idea of health (i.e. a stable state of 'wellness') is a myth, and is merely the person's current (temporary) success in dealing with one of an infinite range of problems in living.

Tidal rejects the traditional idealistic assumptions concerning health (e.g. that health involves the ability to function independently or achieve one's full life potential). Instead, Tidal emphasises that life, for all people, is a continual struggle (although for some that struggle is considerably greater than for others). Everyday life flows and is characterised by flux or instability. As a result, the person is required to address and respond to a wide range of 'problems', which are generated by the instability of everyday life. Some such 'problems' may occur within the person, others will stem from the wider socio-cultural environment and many (arguably the majority) will be interpersonal, involving discrete relationships with other persons.

In the psychiatric/mental health field almost 400 forms of 'psychiatric disorder' are represented in the current edition of the *Diagnostic and Statistical Manual* (American Psychiatric Association, 2000). These 'disorders' are commonly referred to (by professional and lay persons alike) as 'mental illness', 'mental health problems' or 'mental health difficulties' and become, for many, the focus of their practice. Although knowledge about mental illness might be interesting, it is not essential to the task of enabling recovery. Instead, we endorse the view popularised, 70 years ago, by Harry Stack Sullivan that what is called 'mental illness/disorder/difficulty' is a problem in living, experienced as a function of the person living her/his life. (Evans, 1996). These involve problems in relating to self, others or life (and its various challenges) in general. The challenge for the Tidal practitioner is to help the person address, recover from or otherwise deal with such problems in living.

Tidal assumes that even when physically 'ill' or 'unhealthy', people can, nevertheless, display positive ways of living, which might encourage others to assume that the person is healthy or well: the most extreme example being a person's 'living into death', when the body is breaking down through some terminal physical disorder. Experiencing terminal cancer near the end of his life, Shoma Morita used to wheel himself around his neighbourhood picking up pieces of litter. To those who said that a sick professor should not be picking up trash, he replied: 'I am just doing what needs to be done.'

Nursing

Trephotaxis

Proposition 3: The proper focus of nursing must involve the provision of care, which ultimately enables the person's growth and development.

Tidal does not support talk about 'treatment', 'clinical techniques' or the application of so-called 'therapeutic interventions', since these are too closely associated with a narrow medical paradigm, and are relatively new concepts, historically speaking. Instead, Tidal emphasies the virtue of reclaiming, and developing further, the traditional concept of nursing. 'Nursing, as an enduring human, interpersonal activity involved a focus on the promotion of growth and development, deriving from the Old French (*nurice*) and Latin (*nutrire*) to nourish' (Barker, 1999: 103).

Nurses need to 'nourish' the persons in their care in a complete sense, e.g. emotionally, spiritually and intellectually, not just in terms of food and drink. This remains, arguably, the distinctive professional role of the nurse in any setting. In a similar way to the 'nursing/nurturing' provided by parents, the objective is for people to be able to 'grow out' of the need for nursing and to make their own way in the world.

Given the tragic history of psychiatric nurses' institutional/custodial 'care' of people with 'mental illness' (Whitaker, 2003), Tidal proposes that it is vital to affirm the enabling/developmental basis of nursing, if the mistakes of the past are not to be repeated. The shadow of that 'institutional' history remains evident in Halter's (2008) study, which confirmed that psychiatric nurses are still viewed as less 'skilled, logical, dynamic and respected'. Consequently, Tidal proposes that mental health nursing must be based on trephotaxis: 'the provision of the necessary conditions for the promotion of growth and development' (Barker, 1989). Nurses help people, first, to describe and name their experiences in their own language, rather than in the language of nursing, medicine or psychology. This leads to exploring how people might begin better to deal with, if not completely resolve, their problems in living, on their terms. This means that the resultant 'nursing action' will be highly specific to the individual 'person-in-care'.

Tidal assumes that nursing is neither science nor art. The proper focus of nursing is to develop a 'craft' (Barker and Whitehill, 1997). The meaning of any act of caring is not determined by the nurse who delivers it, but by the person who receives it. Nurses need to develop skills and knowledge, which are similar to the technical (scientific) and aesthetic (art) skills of a jeweller or potter. However, ultimately the meaning (value) attached to the piece of jewellery or pottery is attributed by the person who owns the piece (Barker, 2009).

Environment

A world of relations

Proposition 4: The person is involved in an continual, interactive relationship with the world of experience, within which the person creates a sense of 'self' and 'others'.

The physical and socio-cultural worlds exert obvious influences on the growth and development of the individual person. Most people learn how to take shelter from the elements; some people learn how to encourage others to offer them refuge; but only a few develop original ways of protecting themselves or their loved ones from an inhospitable world.

Read and Hammersley (2006) have drawn a provocative link between one example of an 'inhospitable world', childhood trauma (sexual abuse, etc.), and the development of 'psychosis' in adulthood. However, not all children who experience such childhood trauma develop a 'psychosis' or any other form of 'mental illness'. This suggests that children who ultimately are given a diagnosis of schizophrenia may have developed a particular relationship with their early experience, which ultimately proved to be psychologically debilitating. Certainly, the use of the term 'psychological' means to reduce or resolve aspects of 'psychosis', such as 'hearing voices', suggesting that the person's relationship with events, even from the distant past, can be modified significantly.

Tidal acknowledges that the problems in living, which are ultimately described as 'mental illness', have their discrete origins in the interpersonal and intrapersonal worlds, where discrete experiences within the physical, social and cultural environments, are transformed into stories, which serve to identify who the person is, and what they are becoming.

Tidal language

Metaphor and meaning

In Goatley's (1997: 336) view: 'Language is more metaphorical, less literal than we are accustomed to think.' The English language, in particular, is awash with metaphors, especially with metaphors of nautical origin. Britain's high coastline to population ratio helps to explain how maritime metaphors shaped the English language. However, the sea and the way it shapes the land, has a special metaphorical meaning. Fry (2008) suggested: 'Language is shaped, like a coastline, by a flow of metaphors, which erode, break down and eventually become part of everyday speech and writing.'

Tidal acknowledges that change (like the sea) is the only constant in all our lives: rhythmic in nature, and ebbing and flowing like the tide. The experience of change in both breakdown and recovery often 'comes and goes'; or is like 'two steps forward, one back'. Nautical metaphors are commonly used to describe uncertain or dramatic states, e.g. drifting, washed up, wrecked or drowning.

Traditionally people with problems in living have been encouraged to think of themselves as being in some fixed state, e.g. 'I am an alcoholic' or 'I have schizophrenia'. Tidal recognises that all human experience is ephemeral, ebbing and flowing like the tide. Sometimes a person is like 'this' and at other times, like 'that'. The experience of 'breakdown' and 'recovery' often seems to 'come and go'; 'two steps forward, one step back'. Most languages have nautical metaphors to describe such uncertain or dramatic states. Tidal practitioners seek to discover and employ the person's own preferred metaphors, thus respecting the language the person uses to tell her or his own unique story.

Life as narrative and narrative-based practice

Tidal's emphasises a form of discourse, which differs markedly from the 'methods' of evidence-based nursing practice. Narrative is always about particular human instances, whereas evidence-based practice is based on the behaviour of populations, whose elements are merely assumed to be equivalent. Tidal's story focus is not concerned to unravel the 'cause' of the person's present problems of living but, instead, aims to use the experience of the person's journey and its associated meanings to chart the 'next step' that needs to be taken on the person's life voyage.

Recording the narrative

As part of this, in exploring the person's 'world of experience' all records of the Tidal conversations are written entirely in the person's own voice, rather than translated into a third person account, or professional language. The nurse and the person in care co-create a narrative account of the person's experience. This includes the identification of what the person believes is needed at that moment, in terms of nursing care, and holds the promise of what 'needs to happen' to meet that need.

Whatever the so-called 'clinical presentation', Tidal gives precedence to the person's story, since this is the location for the enactment of the person's life: it is the theatre of experience in which reflection and discussion result in a contemporaneous script editing. The caring process (Barker, 2000c) begins and ends here, since all people express a need to develop (or create) a coherent account of what has happened, and what is presently happening to them, in the light of her/his personal experience. When the person is discharged from care, he or she takes home copies of all these 'records' as documentary evidence of that part of the life voyage.

The value base

Philosophical approach

Originally described as a philosophical approach to the development of practice-based evidence in mental healthcare (Barker, 2000a), Tidal invites practitioners to ask how they might tailor care to fit the specific needs of the person and the person's story and unique lived experience, so that the person might begin, or advance further on the voyage of recovery.

The Tidal practitioner's trephotaxic approach expresses six key philosophical assumptions:

- Belief in the virtue of curiosity: the person is the world authority on her/his life and its problems. By expressing genuine curiosity, the professional can learn something of the 'mystery' of the person's story.
- Recognition of the power of resourcefulness: rather than focusing on problems, deficits and weaknesses, Tidal seeks to reveal the many resources available to the person, both personal and interpersonal, that might help on the voyage of recovery.
- Respect for the person's wishes: rather than being paternalistic (suggesting that we might 'know what is best' for the person) the practitioner explores the person's wishes and desires, related to future action.
- Acceptance of the paradox of crisis as opportunity. Challenging events in our lives signal that something 'needs to be done'. This might become an opportunity for change in life direction.
- Acknowledging that all goals must, obviously, belong to the person. These will represent the small steps on the road to recovery.
- The virtue in pursuing elegance. Psychiatric care and treatment is often complex and bewildering. The simplest possible means are sought, which might bring about the changes needed for the person to move forward.

The Tidal commitments

The 10 commitments articulate the core values and also provide a basis for auditing practice. Twenty Tidal 'competencies' (two for each Tidal commitment) have been developed for use in auditing the extent to which an individual practitioner (or team) is enacting the core Tidal philosophy. See www.tidal-model.com. All the practical processes of the Tidal Model are based on the enactment of one or more of the 10 commitments.

1. Value the voice: The person's story represents the beginning and endpoint of the helping encounter, embracing not only an account of the person's distress, but also the hope for its resolution. The story is spoken by the voice of experience. We seek to encourage the voice of the person, rather than enforce the voice of authority.

Traditionally, the person's story is 'translated' into a third person professional account, by different health or social care practitioners. This becomes not so much the person's story (my story) but the professional team's view of that story (history). Tidal seeks to help people develop their unique narrative accounts into a formalised version of 'my story', through ensuring that all Tidal records are written in the person's own 'voice'. If the person is unable, or unwilling, to write, then the nurse acts as secretary, recording what has been agreed, conjointly; writing this in the 'voice' of the person.

2. Respect the language: People develop unique ways of expressing their life stories, representing to others that which only they can know. The language of the story, complete with its unusual grammar and personal metaphors, is the ideal medium for illuminating the way to recovery. We encourage people to speak their own words in their distinctive voice.

Traditionally, stories written about 'patients' by professionals are framed by the arcane, technical language of psychiatric medicine or psychology. Regrettably, many service users and consumers often learn to describe themselves in the colonial language of the professionals who have diagnosed them (Buchanan-Barker and Barker, 2002). By valuing and using the person's natural language, the Tidal practitioner conveys the simplest, yet most powerful, respect for the person.

3. Develop genuine curiosity: The person is writing a life story but is in no sense an 'open book'. No one can know another person's experience. Consequently, professionals need to express genuine interest in the story so that they can better understand the storyteller and the story.

Often, professionals are only interested in 'what is wrong' with the person, or in pursuing particular lines of professional inquiry, for example, seeking 'signs and symptoms' or 'nursing diagnoses'. Genuine curiosity reflects an interest in the person and the person's unique experience, as opposed to merely classifying and categorising features, which might be common to many other 'patients'.

4. Become the apprentice: The person is the world expert on the life story. Professionals may learn something of the power of that story, but only if they apply themselves diligently and respectfully to the task by becoming apprentice-minded. We need to learn from the person, what needs to be done, rather than leading.

Professionals often talk as if they might even know people better than they know themselves. As Szasz noted: 'How can you know more about a person after seeing him for a few hours, a few days or even a few months, than he knows about himself? He has known himself a lot longer. ...The idea that the person remains entirely in charge of himself is a fundamental premise' (Szasz, 2000).

5. Use the available toolkit: The person's story contains examples of 'what has worked' for the person in the past or beliefs about 'what might work' for this person in the future. These represent the main 'tools' that need to be used to unlock or build the story of recovery. The professional toolkit, commonly expressed through ideas such as 'evidence-based practice', describes only what has 'worked' for other people (usually 'research subjects').

6. Craft the step beyond: The professional helper and the person work together to construct an appreciation of what needs to be done 'now'. Any 'first step' is a crucial step, revealing the power of change and potentially pointing towards the ultimate goal of recovery. Lao Tzu said that the journey of a thousand miles begins with a single step. We would go further: any journey begins in our imagination. It is important to imagine, or envision, moving forward. Crafting the step beyond reminds us of the importance of working with the person in the 'me now': addressing what needs to be done now, to help advance to the next step.

7. Give the gift of time: Although time is largely illusory, nothing is more valuable. Time is the midwife of change. Often, professionals complain about not having enough time to work constructively with the person. Although they may not actually 'make' time, through creative attention to their work, professionals often find the time to do 'what needs to be done'. Here, it is the professional's relationship with the concept of time, which is at issue, rather than time itself (Jonsson, 2005).

8. Reveal personal wisdom: Only the person can know him or herself. The person develops a powerful storehouse of wisdom through the writing of the life story. Often, people cannot find the words to express fully the magnitude, complexity or ineffability of their experience, invoking powerful personal metaphors to convey something of their experience (Barker, 2002). A key task for the professional is to help the person reveal and come to value that wisdom, so that it might be used to sustain the person throughout the voyage of recovery.

9. Know that change is constant: Change is inevitable for change is constant. This is the common story for all people. However, decisions have to be made if growth is to occur. The nurse's task is to develop awareness of how change is happening now, and to support the person in making decisions regarding the course of the recovery voyage.

10. Be transparent: If the person and the professional helper are to become a team then each must put down their 'weapons'. In the story-writing process the professional's pen can all too often become a weapon: writing a story that risks inhibiting, restricting and delimiting the person's life choices. Professionals are in a privileged position and should model confidence by being transparent at all times; helping the person understand exactly what is being done and why. By retaining the use of the person's own language, and by completing all records together (in situ), the collaborative nature of the professional–person relationship becomes even more transparent.

Domains of personhood

The world of experience

Tidal views the experience of mental distress as a drama: there are few more dramatic life events than the prospect or experience of 'losing one's mind' (in popular parlance). The organisation and delivery of mental health services becomes part of the personal drama of psychiatric breakdown and

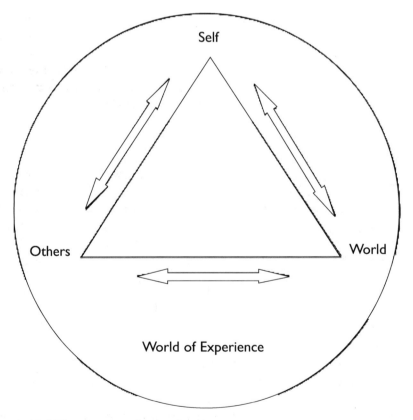

Figure 10.1. The domains of personhood.

recovery. Although the idea that mental healthcare is primarily a 'scientific' venture is popular, the help people need more often resembles the drama of traditional literature. The experience of madness (or mental illness, mental health problem, psychiatric disorder) and our various attempts to respond to the person's distress, whether as professionals, family or friends, often are highly 'dramatic'. Some of our colleagues with experience of 'psychotic disorders' have encouraged us to revive this expression, thus reclaiming use of a term once used to disempower people (see Barker et al, 1999)

Husserl and Heidegger's idea of the lived world or lifeworld (McCann, 1993) refers to the universe within which we live, but which is experienced (or perceived) differently by each of us. All individuals have their own individual perspective on the world, framed by what is often called their 'outlook' or 'point of reference'. Once we begin to analyse, name and (especially) talk about some of the things we experience, and the context within which these experiences are set, we begin to unfold a narrative. In time, this becomes part of the story of our experience, representing our personal view of the 'lifeworld' and our actions within it.

Tidal asserts that the person's whole lived experience, the story, is central to the unfolding drama of breakdown and recovery, and is channelled through three distinct but inter-related domains which represent a metaphorical 'living space' within the person – self, world and others (see *Figure 10.1*). These represent dimensions of the person's overall relationship to the theatre of experience. They are the metaphorical settings for the action of the person's story.

The self domain

The self domain represents the most private aspect of the person: the emotional hinterland, from which people view the action of their stories as they develop within the world domain. The self domain is the place where people feel their lives in progress. Much of this is beyond words (arguably it is pre-linguistic) but can be expressed through metaphor, simile or 'feeling talk'.

The crisis that first brought the person into contact with the mental health services, first makes its mark in the self domain. Here people feel the effects of the problem of living, and become aware of the threat it poses to their identity or well-being. In practical terms the self domain is the place where people need the most sensitive support. Nurses aim to facilitate the conditions that might represent the 'safe haven' that individuals need to begin the necessary repair work on the story of their life.

The practical work of the professional team within the self domain is focused on facilitating a sense of security, both physical and emotional, through the development of a personal security plan. Details of all the processes in the Tidal Model, such as the personal security plan, holistic assessment, and groupwork are provided alongside illustrations from practice in the *Tidal Model Manual* (available from: www.tidal-model.com). This focuses on nurturing the person's sense of security in very practical terms; defining the role of the person and others in facilitating this state.

The world domain

In the world domain the person begins to bring out into the world some aspects of the private story located within the self domain. This is done through talking and writing about such 'private' experiences. The holistic assessment (described in detail later) provides one means for helping the person begin to tell the story of what is happening now within the 'world of experience' and how this relates to memories of past events; and begin to explore the personal meaning of this story. This leads, eventually, to exploring the kind of support that might be needed to address the issues raised by this story.

Although much has been written about the perceived need for holistic mental healthcare, few practical examples exist of how this might be realised. The holistic assessment offers one theoretically supported, flexible template for setting the person's problems into a genuine 'real-life' context.

This conversation is developed further within one-to-one sessions, which focus on helping the person identify and discuss current issues, problems or difficulties; identifying what the person might do, and what help might be received from others, to begin to address them.

The others domain

The others domain deals with the person's relationship with the social world, and the interpersonal support that might be available.

Three forms of group work aim to help people reclaim their personal power and identify personal and interpersonal resources. These processes strengthen social cohesion and rehearse the community affiliations vital to social survival in the natural community.

- The discovery group helps people become more aware of personal aspects of life experience, which have shaped (or are shaping) who and what they are, as persons.
- The information sharing group helps people learn more about specific services, issues or other topics, which they have chosen to explore.
- The solutions group helps people become more aware of how they can draw support and encouragement from their peers who are 'in the same boat' as themselves.

These groups help to build a sense of community, which hopefully will act as a bridge to supportive communities in the natural social world.

Reclaiming the psyche

Tidal assumes that the person's mental distress has emerged as a function of life experience in the world of the natural community. Psychiatry originally meant (in Latin) the 'curing of the soul' or (in Old French) the 'healing care of the mind'. The emphasis on the mind is peculiar to only some languages, such as English. In German, for example, there is no 'mind', only geist (spirit). In dealing with the 'whole person', as opposed to a discrete, isolated 'illness' or 'disorder', nursing practice needs to take account of all that individuals might be, including their essential spirit or personal identity (Barker and Buchanan-Barker, 2003).

It is assumed that nurses will care about the people in their care, acknowledging their core humanity and, when appropriate, will care for people; helping them to fulfil personal and inter-personal activities that they are unable to fulfil unaided. However, Tidal emphasises caring with the person: developing a constructive, collaborative dialogue of care (Barker and Whitehill, 1997). In 'caring with' people who may be highly distressed, in some 'altered state', suicidal or otherwise 'self-destructive', nurses face significant challenges to their own personal identity, and require considerable support from professional colleagues, usually through sophisticated group or individual supervision.

The key Tidal processes

If the person is to recover her or his life, then the necessary work of recovery must begin as soon as possible: preferably the moment the person connects with the service. Traditionally, a person referred to a service comes accompanied by a referral letter and perhaps a lengthy set of 'case notes'. These represent the professional (hi)story of the 'patient'.

- The first task for the nurse is to find out who is the person behind all these histories, and what problems in living have brought him or her into care?
- Next, the nurse must negotiate with the person the kind of support needed to help begin to address these problems in living.
- Finally, the nurse must negotiate the conditions which will promote the person's sense of personal security. What will help him or her feel more secure and less at risk of harm from self or others?

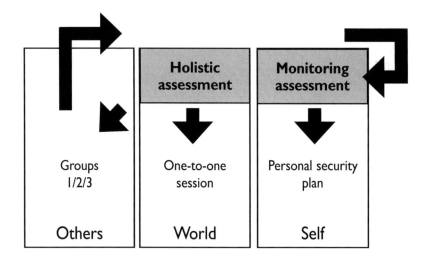

Figure 10.2. The Tidal process from entry to exit.

Different Tidal processes are used to address these issues, but all seek to keep the individuals 'in the driving seat', maintaining their autonomy as far as possible. All Tidal care is seen as a rehearsal for 'self-management'. At some point, individuals will be 'discharged' from care, and will be expected to fend for themselves. No time should be wasted in preparing them for the 'self-management' role they will enter on discharge from the service.

The overall Tidal process from entry to exit is illustrated in *Figure 10.2*. This is highly flexible and, depending on the person's presentation, the 'work' may begin in any of the three domains.

- If people are reluctant to engage in individual work, they may be encouraged to sit in on one of the groups, to become 'acclimatised', and hopefully gain confidence in the team, through exploring the others domain.
- If the person is highly disturbed/disturbing, the initial focus may need to be on developing a personal security plan, exploring the 'threats' that lie deep within the self domain.
- If the person is not a major risk to him or herself or others, the team may begin in the world domain, encouraging the person to begin to tell the story, through the holistic assessment, following this up with dedicated one-to-one sessions, where 'hot issues' of the day, are addressed.

Case study

Dick's story

Here the story of Dick Smith (all details have been changed to protect Dick's identity) is used to illustrate the voyage through care. Dick has a long history of drug and alcohol use, and has had several episodes of hospitalisation for 'psychotic breakdowns'. Five days ago he attempted suicide by jumping into a river from a bridge. Following rescue, he spent three days in medical care before being transferred to the psychiatric unit. Dick is reluctant to talk and has, in the past, been described as 'non-compliant'.

The personal security plan

On entry to the service, the team needs to find out who Dick is and what has brought him into its care. First however, the team must try to help him feel as safe and secure as possible.

Despite being reluctant to talk, the primary nurse, Kit (although a range of team members is involved, Kit is used here to represent 'the team'), focuses on developing with Dick a highly provisional personal security plan. Psychiatric services often focus on 'safety': managing the physical and social environment so that any risk of harm is minimised. However, the 'risk' lies within the person's self domain – not in the outside world. 'Safety precautions' are important, but do not address the issue of 'personal insecurity'. Through discussion, the nurse hopes that Dick will help her appreciate what Dick might be able to do, and what the professional team might do, to help him feel at least a little more secure. If the person is reluctant to engage with the personal security plan, the team will do all it can to make the person 'safe', while it continues to try to engage the person in developing the personal security plan.

Kit: I know that you have been having rough time. I'd like to talk with you about how we could make things as comfortable here for you as possible. OK?
Dick: [Says nothing.]
Kit: I guess that you can't really be bothered with any of this, but it is important for me, and my colleagues, to know what sorts of things might make you feel better, within yourself.
Dick: [Says nothing.]
Kit: Well, I don't know how you are feeling right now, and maybe you don't really want to tell me, but I guess if I am to be of any help to you, I need you to give me some pointers. I know what helps me, and I could tell you, but right now I really would like to know what helps you. Can we talk about that?

This conversation begins to rehearse the collaborative relationship, which will be threaded through all the other Tidal interactions, involving the nursing team. For many people used to standard psychiatric practice, such 'openness' can be fairly threatening. Kit's challenge is to help Dick appreciate that she is being transparent (rather than trying to manipulate him), and that she genuinely wants to learn from him, about what would help right now. Needless to say, this requires the nurse to have some (perhaps considerable) interpersonal skills. To assume that anyone could do this, seems foolhardy.

As Kit gains Dick's confidence, they begin to map out, simply, the kind of things that Dick could do to 'help him feel more safe and secure', and the kind of things that 'others might do to help him feel more secure'. As they talk, Kit makes a note of the points they are discussing (Dick sees this as 'the nurse's job, anyway'). At the end of the session, Kit makes a copy, and encourages Dick to keep this to refer to as a memory aid, trying out the plan as part of his everyday routine. This will be revised and adapted over the succeeding days, as 'useful' things are maintained or developed further, and 'ineffective' things are dropped and replaced by alternatives. Since all such 'notes' are confidential, Kit discusses with Dick how he might keep his private belongings safe.

The monitoring assessment

Over the succeeding days, Kit and her colleagues gain more of Dick's confidence and they begin to use the monitoring assessment, as a means of helping Dick to reflect on himself, his feelings, and the developing relationship with the nursing team.

- Kit begins the session by inviting Dick to talk about how he is feeling, or more generally, asks, 'How are you doing?' A note about these feeling is made (by Dick or the nurse) in Dick's own words.
- Dick is encouraged to reflect on how this feeling affects him, in terms of feeling 'safe' or 'vulnerable'. Usually a scale is used to help Dick 'step back' from (or externalise) the feeling. Alternatively he could represent its effect with a drawing.
- Dick is encouraged to talk more about, and make notes on 'what helps' at the moment.
- If appropriate, the nurse invites Dick to think about the chances of coming to harm (or harming someone else, if that is more appropriate). This brings any 'risk' issues out into the open where they can be discussed more honestly and directly. Although some people find this uncomfortable, most people express relief that they can at last talk openly about their fears, especially related to self-harm, suicide or anger and resentment towards others.

- Dick is asked to judge to what extent he thinks that Kit (or any other team member or other person) could help him feel 'more secure'. Again, a rating (or drawing) helps Dick 'stand back' from (or externalise) the issue. These 'ratings' are merely a device to accentuate Dick's 'relationship' with thoughts and feelings.
- Dick has already talked about what appears to 'work' for him right now. What has he thought about, but never tried? What has he heard others talk about, or read about, that he might consider trying for himself?
- Kit asks Dick to judge (with a rating) to what extent he feels confident that he can keep himself safe, until the next session.
- Finally, Kit asks herself the same question (aloud), reflecting on her view of Dick's situation. If there is a discrepancy between Dick's rating of 'confidence' and that of the nurse, the nurse invites Dick to talk about this; to reflect on why there might be a difference of opinion. This encourages Dick to empathise with the nurse – and perhaps consider his situation through someone else's eyes. There is no need, however, to reconcile the difference, only to discuss it.

Again, a copy of the notes is made for Dick's own reference and safe-keeping and the original placed in his records.

The holistic assessment

The holistic assessment is a five-page template for exploring, in more detail, aspects of Dick's 'lifeworld'; especially the problems in living that brought Dick into care. After providing a simple rationale for the session, Kit asks Dick, 'What has brought you here?' or 'How have you come to be here, now'. (N.B. Kit does not ask Dick to talk about his 'problems' far less his 'illness/disorder'. He may believe that he has no such problems/illness.)

Once Dick has identified an issue, difficulty or other 'problem in living' (something, he either wishes, or needs, to talk about), Kit begins to explore this in detail. What follows represents only the basic line of inquiry. Kit will ask additional questions, and summarise her understanding of Dick's answers, to promote a sense of 'conversation'.

- *Problem origins:* 'When did you first become aware of this "problem" or "difficulty"? What was going on in your life around that time?'
- *Past problem function:* 'How did this problem (issue, etc.) affect you, in the beginning? How did it affect the everyday living of your life?'

- *Past emotional context*: 'How did you feel about that (what has just been described) at the time?'
- *Historical development*: 'In what way have things changed over time, for you?'
- *Relationships*: 'What effect has all of this had (what Dick is talking about) on the people in your life?' Although written by Kit, the responses are in Dick's own voice.
- *Current emotional context*: 'Given all that you have said, how do you feel about all of this now, at this very moment?'
- *Holistic content*: Kit summarises the story so far using Dick's words carefully. 'When you think about all of this what does this mean, for you, like personally? What's it all about, Dick?'
- *Holistic context:* 'What do you think that this (what has been discussed) says about you as a person?'
- *Needs, wants and wishes:* 'What do you hope might be done to begin to address these problems/issues?'
- *Expectations:* 'What do you expect that I might do to help you with any of this, or anyone else for that matter?'
- *Evaluation*: Dick might wish to talk about his 'problem/issues' as one whole thing, or he might split these up into different parts or separate 'problems'. Using a simple rating scale Dick is asked to rate :
  - 'How much distress does this "thing" (or these separate problems) cause you?'
  - 'To what extent do they disturb or upset the everyday living of your life?'
  - 'What control, if any, do you have over them?'
- *Personal resources*: Although help and support is being offered by the team, Dick must spend much of his time alone with his problems. Certainly, when he is discharged, he will spend almost all of his time alone with his problems. In anticipation of this situation, Dick is encouraged to reflect on his personal and interpersonal sources of support.
  - 'Tell me a bit about the people, things or beliefs you have about life in general, that are important to you? Let's begin with people. Who is important to you in your life? Can you tell me why this person is important to you?'
- *Resolution*: The final stage of the holistic assessment prepares the ground for the one-to-one sessions which will follow. 'How will you know when [whatever Dick has been talking about] is no longer a problem/issue for you? What do you think needs to happen [or to change] for you to begin to deal with this [problem/issue]?'

Finally, Kit makes a copy of the holistic assessment for Dick, putting the original in his notes, for reference by the rest of the team. The record format is split into two columns. The left-hand column addresses issues for Dick; the left-hand column addresses (mainly) issues for the team to consider and act upon. This side-by-side format further tries to illustrate (graphically) the collaborative nature of the relationship.

One-to-one sessions

Over the next few days Kit and her colleagues spend more time with Dick in one-to-one sessions. A record of these conversations is also made, in Dick's own words and he is encouraged to keep a copy as a reminder of what he needs to do to deal with his problems.

- Kit opens the session by asking Dick, 'What's on your mind or otherwise troubling you?'. With much support and prompting Dick says: 'I've never liked myself. I'm bad. I'm a sinner.'
- Kit asks him how he 'would want it to be'. This becomes Dick's ultimate 'aim'. For many people this 'aim' might appear a very remote possibility. However, this is an important destination on the person's recovery voyage. Every effort is made to make this 'aim' as concrete as possible. With much prompting Dick says that he would like to 'be more positive about myself', adding 'but I know that will never happen'. Kit suggests they write: 'Be more positive about myself' adding, 'Let's wait, and see if that happens. What do you think?'
- Kit asks Dick to talk about when he last 'didn't feel too bad about himself – at least a little bit less bad.' He talks about being out walking that morning.
- Kit asks him to go into detail about what exactly he was doing when out walking.
- Kit summarises what Dick has said and then asks him what he might be able to do with this. With some support and further questioning, Dick says, 'Maybe I should do more stuff.' (His mother always said to him that 'idle hands make work for the devil'.)
- Kit then asks what he thinks he should do next, in the next few hours. It is important to translate the reflections into action as soon as possible.
- Moving to the team's side of the record, she asks Dick to tell her what she (and other team members) could do to help him carry out this plan.
- Then she asks how he feels about the support he is getting (in general) on the unit. 'What's helpful? What do you find unhelpful?'

- Moving towards the conclusion, Kit asks Dick to help her summarise what they have been talking about in the session.
- Finally, she asks Dick: 'How did you find this session?'

The one-to-one sessions are based entirely on Dick's rolling agenda: what is important changes from day to day. Dick also has a 'problem list' which details his physical health problems, finances and certain legal issues, with which he may need additional help or support. These are, however, separate from the 'flowing' problems in living, which need to be addressed from day to day. Over time, Dick learns that issues crop up that he needs to address, but some of these he tries to avoid. In time, he gains confidence to address the issues and problems that he has previously avoided. The Tidal 'care continuum' acknowledges that as people progress, the focus of the care needed can become 'deeper' – exploring problems of living in more depth or at greater length (see Barker and Buchanan-Barker, 2005: 44–50).

Group work

With some encouragement, Dick joins the discovery group that Kit and Jenny are facilitating.

This group uses a variety of formats to encourage the members to talk about themselves as people, rather than 'patients'. All talk about 'illness' or 'problems' is 'off limits'. The two nurses who facilitate also answer some of the questions and their (selective) self-disclosure helps the group members see them as people, with lives (and feelings) of their own. The group is highly supportive – a model for the natural supportive community, most people value.

Dick enjoys listening to the other people talk about the things that are important in their life, their hopes and dreams, and the obstacles they have overcome. Although he does not speak, he feels quite emotional afterwards. The mix of laughter and poignant stories was a new experience for him: 'Not like any other therapy group I've been in'.

Later, Dick joins a solutions group, where Tommy talks about his 'voices' and how he cannot get any relief.

The solutions group has one facilitator, who encourages a 'volunteer' to talk about a 'problem or issue'. Then the group members are encouraged to learn more about the person by asking questions. The 'volunteer' is 'in the driving seat' at all times, and is under no pressure to answer. After several rounds of questions, if the volunteer is willing, the group is encouraged to make comments, suggestions, or otherwise 'bear witness' to the problem under discussion. Before concluding, the facilitator summarises the discussion and asks the volunteer, 'What is different now, compared with when you first started talking?'

Dick feels a great sympathy for Tommy: 'I know what you're talking about.' He discusses with Tommy his experience of 'voices'. Other members ask them both questions, and afterwards Dick tells Kit, 'I felt useful. I haven't felt useful in a long time.'

The solutions group aims to help the members develop their awareness that the beginnings of many of the 'answers' they seek lie either in their own hands, or may be found among friends, family or others who are 'in the same boat'.

Finally, Dick attended the information-sharing group several times over the last two week of his stay. He and some other people asked for information about support available in the community, and a member of the community team, along with two representatives from mutual-support projects, came along to answer questions. Dick enjoyed this group. 'I didn't feel that we were being talked down to. We could ask whatever we liked. I learned a lot.'

Evaluation

When discharged back to the care of the community team, three things made a difference for Dick.

- He said would never have started to talk about his voices and the way people scared him, if Kit had not kept coming back, over and over again. At first, Dick could not understand why she wanted to know what was happening for him. 'Usually,' he said, 'they [nurses and doctors] only want to talk about my illness and stuff.'
- He always knew that the doctors and nurses wrote things about him, but he had never seen what they had written. At first he was unnerved by Kit's willingness to share what she was writing with him, and to make copies for him to take away for reference. This took a lot of getting used to. 'Gradually, I realised Kit was right. This is my life. It's all about me!'
- When an old friend came to see him, he was able to show him the copies of the records of the sessions. 'When I got visits before, people would say, "What you been doing?", and I could never remember.' When discharged, Dick took home a file of his copies of the sessions, along with other notes he had made in a journal. 'Last time I went home, all I had was an appointment card!'

Conclusion

Tidal has been described by at least one user/consumer as the 'beginnings of self-management' (Whitehill, 2005). As noted previously, we believe that the fundamental aim of nursing, as a social activity, is to help people grow and develop, and ultimately fend for themselves as much as possible. Regrettably, some 'recovery models' emphasise the 'self-management' work to the exclusion of any consideration of the contribution made through the conjoint (nursing) work with members of the professional team.

We have collected many stories about the experience of Tidal . However, unsolicited comments can be more revealing, as the following example from a young woman from North America shows:

> *When my nurse first introduced me to the Tidal Model I didn't like it at all. I thought it was too formal and didn't like her writing down the things I said. I saw her a week ago and we were remembering that time. I recognised that my thoughts toward the Tidal Model have changed. And if I look honestly, I have accomplished more since starting with the Tidal Model than I have in my entire life…it's more about what has changed 'inside'. I almost can't believe that this thing I despised is one of the things that helped me the most. I feel like my own voice is heard. I feel empowered and that we work as a team. I feel like she is interested in things I have to say and she helps me see the change and work that has taken place. I am aided in taking the actions necessary to make those changes and my experience is never argued against. We look at what has worked and when I can't see things, she is able to point them out to me.*
>
> *I feel like the Tidal Model has made room for my voice. I'm not just another patient who is mentally ill. I am a person with goals and dreams and a life worth living. I want to thank you for giving me, and hopefully many others, that voice. I get to discover and learn and make changes all the time. Now I know that I can think, decide and act for myself. I don't need someone else to save me any more, because you have given me the opportunity to save myself.*

'Self-management' must begin at the point of entry into the service, not at the point of discharge. The recovery voyage must begin at the nadir or lowest poin, literally 'the point beneath our feet'. Through this work individuals begin to rehearse their story of the kind of decisions and actions that might be needed as part of everyday living, once returned to ordinary life in the community. This work is rarely easy for the nurse, far less for the person in care.

The young woman featured in the quote above said that she wanted to thank us for 'giving her back her voice'. We thanked her for her generosity, but noted that it was not us she should thank, but rather the nurse who persisted in working with her. She agreed.

Her story reminds us that, like all other 'models' and 'theories', the Tidal Model does not work, only individual nurses or teams might 'work' in enabling recovery, although Tidal might help them work out how to do that work.

Ultimately, however, the model and its underpinning theory and philosophy are merely ideas on paper. Those ideas need people to bring them to life, like the persistent, obviously skilled nurse who helped this young woman.

The concept of recovery has gained a degree of presence in the mental health nursing literature (e.g. Jones et al, 2008; Jensen and Wadkins, 2007), although for various philosophical and political reasons it remains problematic (Craig, 2008). The same might be said of the emergence of the concept of 'mental health nursing'. The often contested ideology underpinning the shift from 'psychiatric' to 'mental health' nursing is, however, often fudged by simply marrying these distinct titles: e.g. psychiatric/mental health nursing.

In Cutcliffe and Ward's (2006) view much confusion remains over what psychiatric/mental health nursing is. Despite 20 years discussion of the 'proper focus' of nursing in psychiatric/mental healthcare (Barker, 1989; 1999), in most countries the discipline continues to be shaped and steered by largely anonymous bureaucracies, which express the political agendas of the Government in office. However, 'nursing' as a social activity existed long before it acquired the restrictive definition associated with the professional discipline (Barker, 1989; 1999).

Morrall (2006) may have been accurate in observing that the contemporary discourse of psychiatric/mental health nursing pivots around social control. However, how things 'are' bears no relationship to how things 'ought' to be. Such 'social controllers' may be called nurses, but they are not practising 'nursing'; at least not in a way recognisable to linguists, far less to lay people who have not learned the arcane language of healthcare.

It is all too apparent that a sizeable body of people called 'psychiatric/ mental health nurses' are unhappy with the expectation that they should merely be agents of social control; many wish to nurture, once again, the idea of nursing as a 'nourishing', 'enabling' activity. The Tidal Model of recovery and reclamation might represent one means by which nurses might recover nursing by reclaiming their nurturing birthright.

Applications and measures of the Tidal Model in practice

- Berger (2006): This paper illustrates of the use of the Tidal Model within a broad-based clinical programme.
- Brookes et al (2006): This is a description of the first introduction of the Tidal Model within a range of clinical settings in North America.
- Lafferty and Davidson (2006): This is a description of the first introduction of the Tidal Model within acute psychiatric care in Scotland and its relationship with the 'rights-based principles' of the Scottish Mental Health Act.

Empirical papers that use the Tidal Model as the theoretical underpinning

- Stevenson et al (2002): This article is a description of the development of the original evaluation protocol for the Tidal Model in England. This has been used as the basis for most of subsequent empirical evaluations of the Tidal Model in other countries.
- Gordon et al (2004): This detailed report describes the development and implementation of the Tidal Model within one acute psychiatric ward in Birmingham, England. It also includes details of the comparison of the Tidal ward and four other similar acute wards over a three-year period.
- Cook et al (2005): This research report is on the perceptions of staff and people in forensic care to the introduction of the Tidal Model in New Zealand.
- Gordon et al (2005): This evaluation report is on the introduction of the Tidal Model within acute psychiatric care in England.

Suggested further reading: Theoretical comparisons and explorations of the Tidal Model

A full list of Tidal publications is available at http://www.tidal-model.com/ Tidal%20Ref%20List.%20htm.htm

- Barker (2001): This paper describes how the Tidal Model extends and develops traditional assumptions concerning the centrality of interpersonal relations within nursing practice, emphasising in particular the importance of perceived meanings within the lived experience of the person-in-care and the role of the narrative in the development of person-centred care plans.
- Fletcher and Stevenson (2001): This article gives a description of the original pilot study within which the Tidal Model was introduced into two wards in the acute mental health services in Newcastle City Health Trust, England
- Stevenson and Fletcher (2002): This is a Royal College of Nursing Continuous Professional Development Series paper which describes in detail the development and practice of the Tidal Model.
- Barker and Buchanan-Barker (2004a): This article discusses the role of mental health nurses in optimising the power of the storyteller as a tool for the person's self-healing. Includes evaluative stories from the Tidal Model.
- Barker and Buchanan-Barker (2004b): This is a description of the development of the interpersonal concept of 'bridging' and its role in

the care of people deemed to be at risk of harm to self or others.

- Barker and Buchanan-Barker (2005) Definitive text on the theory and development of the model and its practice.
- Barker and Buchanan-Barker (2007): This unpublished manual is available as a free PDF download from www.tidal-model.com

References

American Psychiatric Association (2000) *Diagnostic and Statistical Manual of Mental Disorders DSM-IV-TR* 4th edn. American Psychiatric Association, Washington, DC

Barker P (1982) *Behaviour Therapy Nursing*. Croom Helm, London

Barker PJ (1989) Reflections on the philosophy of caring in mental health. *International Journal of Nursing Studies* **26**(2): 131–41

Barker PJ (1990) Needs and wants and fairy-tale wishes: A Scottish impression of care in the community. *Architecture and Comportment: Architecture and Behaviour* **6**(3): 233–44

Barker P (1998) It's time to turn the tide. *Nursing Times* **18**(94): 70–2

Barker P (1999) *The Philosophy and Practice of Psychiatric Nursing*. Churchill Livingstone, Edinburgh

Barker P (2000a) The Tidal Model: The lived experience in person-centred mental healthcare. *Nursing Philosophy* **2**(3): 213–23

Barker P (2000b) Working with the metaphor of life and death. *Journal of Medical Ethics: Medical Humanities* **26**: 97–102

Barker P (2000c) The virtue of caring. *International Journal of Nursing Studies* **37**: 329–36

Barker P (2001) The Tidal Model: The lived experience in person-centred mental healthcare. *Nursing Philosophy* **2**(3): 213–23

Barker P (2002) The Tidal Model: The healing potential of metaphor within the patient's narrative. *Journal of Psychosocial Nursing and Mental Health Services* **40**(7): 42–50

Barker P (2009) *Psychiatric and Mental Health Nursing: The Craft of Caring*. Hodder Arnold, London

Barker P, Buchanan-Barker P (2003) *Spirituality and Mental Health: Breakthrough*. Whurr, London

Barker P, Buchanan-Barker P (2004a) Beyond empowerment: Revering the storyteller. *Mental Health Practice* **7**(5): 18–20

Barker P, Buchanan-Barker P (2004b) Bridging: Talking meaningfully about the care of people at risk. *Mental Health Practice* **8**(3): 12–16

Barker P, Buchanan-Barker P (2005) *The Tidal Model: A Guide forMental Health Professionals*. Brunner-Routledge, London

Barker P, Buchanan-Barker P (2007) *The Tidal Model: Mental Health, Reclamation and Recovery*. Unpublished manual. Available from… www.

tidal-model.com

Barker P, Buchanan-Barker P (2008a) *This Tide's Already Changed.* Available from: http://www.psychminded.co.uk/news/news2008/April08/phil_barker003. htm Accessed 28th August 2008

Barker P, Buchanan-Barker P (2008b) Reclaiming nursing: Making it personal. *Mental Health Practice* **11**(9). 12–6

Barker P, Campbell P, Davidson B (1999) *From the Ashes of Experience: Reflection on Madness, Survival and Growth.* Whur, London

Barker P, Whitehill I (1997) The Craft of Care: Towards collaborative caring in psychiatric nursing. In: Tilley S ed. *The Mental Health Nurse: Views of Practice and Education.* Blackwell Science, Oxford

Bateson G (1973) *Steps to an Ecology of Mind,* Paladin, London

Berger JL (2006) Incorporation of the Tidal Model into the interdisciplinary plan of care - a program quality improvement project. *Journal of Psychiatric and Mental Health Nursing* **13**(4): 464–7

Brookes N (2005) Phil Barker: The Tidal Model of Mental Health Recovery. In AM Tomey MR Alligood Eds. *Nursing Theorists and their Work* (6th Edn) New York, Mosby

Brookes N (in press) Phil Barker: The Tidal Model of Mental Health Recovery. In AM Tomey MR Alligood Eds. *Nursing Theorists and their Work* (6th Edn) New York, Mosby

Brookes N, Murata L, Tansey M (2006) Guiding practice development using the Tidal Commitments. *J Psychiatric and Mental health Nursing* **13**: 460–3

Buchanan-Barker P (2004) Uncommon sense: The Tidal Model of mental health recovery. *Mental Health Nursing* **23** (1) 12–15

Buchanan-Barker P, Barker P (2002) Lunatic language. *Openmind* **115**: 23

Buchanan-Barker P, Barker P (2008) The Tidal Commitments: Extending the value base of recovery. *Journal of Psychiatric and Mental Health Nursing* **15**: 93–100

Cook NR, Phillips BN, Sadler D (2005) The tidal model as experienced by patients and nurses in a regional forensic unit. *Journal of Psychiatric and Mental Health Nursing* **12**(5): 536–40

Craig TKJ (2008) Recovery: Say what you mean and mean what you say. *Journal of Mental Health* **17**(2): 125–8

Cutcliffe JR, Ward MF (2006) *Key Debates in Psychiatric/Mental Health Nursing* Churchill Livingstone, Edinburgh

Evans FB (1996) *Harry Stack Sullivan: Interpersonal Theory and Psychotherapy.* Routledge, London

Fletcher E, Stevenson C (2001) Launching the Tidal Model in an acute psychiatric ward. *Nursing Standard* **15**(49): 33–6

Fry S (2008) *Fry's English Delight.* Available from: http://www.bbc.co.uk/radio4/ arts/frys_english.shtml [Accessed 28th August 2008]

Goatley A (1997) *The Language of Metaphors* London: Routledge

Gordon W, Morton T, Brooks G (2004) *The Tidal Model and the Reform of*

Nursing Practice. (Unpublished report) Available from: http://www.tidal-model.com/THE%20TIDAL%20MODEL%20Birmingham%20Report.htm

Gordon W, Morton T, Brooks G (2005) Launching the Tidal Model: Evaluating the evidence. *Journal of Psychiatric and Mental Health Nursing* **12:** 703–12

Halter MJ (2008) Perceived characteristics of psychiatric nurses: Stigma by association. *Archives of Psychiatric Nursing* **21**(1): 20–6

Jensen LW, Wadkins TA (2007) Mental health success stories: Finding paths to recovery. *Issues in Mental Health Nursing* **28**(4): 325–40

Jones KM, Gray AH, Paleo J, Braden CJ, Lesser J (2008) Community and scholars unifying for recovery. *Issues in Mental Health Nursing* **29**(5): 495–503

Jonsson B (2005) *Ten Thoughts about Time*. Robinson Publishing, London

Kuhn T (1970). *The Structure of Scientific Revolutions* (2nd Edn), University of Chicago Press, Chicago

Lafferty S, Davidson R (2006) Person-Centred Care in Practice An Account of the Experience of Implementing the Tidal Model in an Adult Acute Admission Ward in Glasgow. *Mental Health Today* **March**: 31–4

McCann C (1993) *Four Phenomenological Philosophers: Husserl, Heidegger, Sartre, Merleau-Ponty*. Routledge, London

Menzies-Lyth I (1959) The Functioning of social systems as a defence against anxiety. In I Menzies-Lyth ed. (1988) *Containing Anxiety in Institutions*. Free Association Books, London

Morita M, Kondo A, Levine P, Morita S (1998) *Morita Therapy and the True Nature of Anxiety-Based Disorders (Shinkeishitsu)*. University of New York, Princeton, MJ

Morrall P (2006) Psychiatry and psychiatric nursing in the New World Order. In JR Cutcliffe, MF Ward eds. Key *Debates in Psychiatric/Mental Health Nursing* Churchill Livingstone, Edinburgh

Read J, Hammersley P (2006) 'Can very bad childhoods drive us crazy? Science, ideology and taboo'. In J Johannessen et al eds. *Evolving Psychosis*. Brunner-Routledge, London

Rogers C (1961) *On Becoming a Person: A Therapist's View of Psychotherapy*. Constable, London

Stevenson C, Barker P, Fletcher E (2002) Judgement days: Developing an evaluation for an innovative nursing model. *Journal of Psychiatric and Mental Health Nursing* **9**(3): 271–6

Stevenson C, Fletcher E (2002) The Tidal Model: The questions answered. *Mental Health Practice* **5**(8): 29–38

Szasz TS (2000) Curing the therapeutic state: Thomas Szasz on the medicalisation of American life. Interviewed by Jacob Sullum. *Reason* **July**: 27–34

Vaughn K, Webster D, Oralhood S, Young B (1995) Brief inpatient psychiatric treatment: Finding solutions. *Issues in Mental Health Nursing* 16(6): 519–31

Whitaker R (2003) *Mad in America: Bad Science, Bad Medicine, and the Enduring Mistreatment of the Mentally Ill*. Basic Books, New York

Whitehill I (2005) Foreword. In P Barker, P Buchanan-Barker. *The Tidal Model: A Guide for Mental Health Professionals*. Brunner-Routledge, London

CHAPTER 11

Critiquing nursing models in the era of evidence-informed practice

Introduction

Subsequent to the publication of a number of the 'earlier' nursing models (e.g. Peplau, 1952; Henderson, 1966) several approaches to critiquing and/or evaluating nursing models were proposed and published. It is perhaps more accurate to point out that several of these attempts were concerned with critiquing and evaluating nursing theory per se (see, for example, Dickoff and James, 1968; Fawcett, 1993; Meleis, 1997) rather than being designed specifically to evaluate nursing models. Nevertheless, examination of the relevant extant literature will show that some work exists that is specific to evaluating nursing models (see, for example, Fitzpatrick and Whall, 1989; Cody, 1999; Fawcett, 1989, 2005; Rodgers, 2005). It should be pointed out, however, that while we have a number of reasonably well-developed approaches to testing theory and models in nursing, McKenna (1997: 236) declares,

You may find in most cases many of these theories have not been tested by researchers, the theorists themselves or by those nurses who use them in practice.

With reference to what the authors have included in each of the chapters in this book that focus on a particular model (i.e. *Chapters 4–10*), we can assert with a degree of confidence that McKenna's 1997 statement is still applicable 12 years later. The existing work that focuses on testing (evaluating) each of the nursing models featured in this book either used the model only as the theoretical underpinning to a study, or used the model as a theoretical guide to certain practice development initiatives, or measured one/some proposition or concept contained with a model (e.g. measurement of self-care agency in Orem's 1980 model). This appears to suggest that we have not moved that far forward from findings reported during the 1980s. We return to this point below.

Approaches to evaluating nursing models: Jacqueline Fawcett's contribution

In the opinion of the authors, one nursing scholar who has clearly made important if not seminal contributions to the substantive area of evaluating nursing models is Jacqueline Fawcett. Fawcett (1989: 51) advances a framework for the evaluation of nursing models which, she argues, 'highlights their most important features and is appropriate to their level of abstraction'.

Fawcett's (1989, 2005) framework contains six elements or steps which are listed in *Box 11.1* and each of these is explored in more detail.

Explication of origins

Fawcett (1989; 2005) argued that the beliefs and values of the original author of any given model of nursing will help to identify the philosophical foundations of the model and help to identify special points of emphasis. While the authors of this book are aware that any person can only ever make public a portion of their core values and beliefs, there may still be merit in seeing some of these. According to several authors, people can only ever know a relatively small portion or percentage of their conscious; they can only ever attain a limited degree of self-awareness. For example, in Freud's (1915–1917) early views, he posited the mind as a natural system and declared that the person was not immediately aware of its inner workings, only its output. Furthermore, that this output was the result of a highly complex, although *unconscious,* process (original emphasis). Freud argued that a great deal of our mental activity is unconscious. Similarly, according to Jarrett (1988), Jung used the analogy of an iceberg to describe a person's conscious/unconscious; with the larger portion of the iceberg (the portion below the surface of the water) representing the person's unconscious, and the smaller portion (the portion above the surface) representing the person's consciousness. Further, Jung argued that a person's shadow material, i.e. all

---

Box 11.1: Fawcett's framework for evaluating nursing models: The six elements/steps

- Explication of origins
- Comprehensiveness of content
- Logical congruence
- Generation of theory
- Credibility of conceptual models
- Contributions to the discipline of nursing

---

those aspects of the person that are seen to be undesirable by the person's ego, are in the unconscious. Fawcett (1989, 2005) posits two questions that need to be asked for evaluating this element namely:

- Are the philosophical claims on which the nursing model is based made explicit?
- Are the scholars who influenced the thinking of the author who designed the model acknowledged and supported by references and citations?

Comprehensiveness of content

Fawcett (1989; 2005) declares that this second element is concerned with the depth and breadth of the content. Fawcett's (2005) comments regarding the lack of standardised and/or widely accepted criteria for evaluating nursing models are still accurate and applicable today. For the authors of this book, this is particularly concerning in the contemporary 'age' or 'era of evidence-based or evidence-informed practice' movement. The problem is, and we return to this issue later in this chapter, captured succinctly by Fawcett (2005:16) who states,

> *The propositions of a conceptual (nursing) model are so abstract and general that they are not amenable to direct observation or empirical testing.*

The lack of standardised or widely accepted criteria notwithstanding, the authors of this book concur with Fawcett's (1989, 2005) view and would therefore expect to see some clear statements within the model pertaining to each of the four metaparadigms and how they relate to one another. Accordingly, Fawcett (1989, 2005: 54) puts forward two specific questions that need to be asked when evaluating a nursing model:

- Does the nursing model provide adequate descriptions of all four concepts of nursing's metaparadigms?
- Do the relational propositions of the nursing model completely link the four metaparadigm concepts?

In addition to these 'theoretical' concerns, given that nursing is ultimately a 'practice-orientated discipline' (see Dickoff et al, 1968; Pearson, 1992; Marris and Lowry, 2006), the authors would argue that a nursing model should make a difference in practice. The well-documented difficulties in evaluating ambiguous nursing models notwithstanding, if a nursing model is to have utility and meaning for clinicians, we would argue that the model must influence practice for the better. These are by no means new arguments. Johnson's (1987) remarks underscored this position when she argued that nursing models should,

> *provide philosophical and pragmatic orientations to the service nurses provide to patients.*

Consequently, as valuable and relevant as evaluation questions related to the theoretical content are, questions about the pragmatic and/or practical content are just as necessary. Fawcett (1989, 2005: 54) advances one such question and this is a fine starting point, she states:

- Is the practitioner given sufficient direction to be able to make pertinent observations, decide that an actual or potential need for nursing exists, and prescribe and execute a course of action that achieves the goal specified by a variety of practice situations?

Other questions we would suggest need to be asked might include:

- How is care which is underpinned by a conceptual model of nursing different to care provided that has no such conceptual underpinning?
- What are the differences in outcomes for clients (and their families/ significant others) and for the nurses themselves, when the care delivered is based on a conceptual nursing model?

Logical congruence

Fawcett (2005) pronounces that the third element to evaluate is concerned with the logic of the internal structure of the model and thus the reviewer ought to examine the congruence (similarity) between what the author of the model claims are the philosophical underpinnings and the actual content of the model. Fawcett (2005) continues and points out that this element is particularly important if the model incorporates more than one world view. Indeed, Fawcett adopts a stance that has been characterised as a 'purist stance' (Greene, 2007) with regards to mixing paradigms and argues that these different paradigms/ world views should first be reformed or translated in order to 'ensure just one congruent frame of reference' (Fawcett, 2005: 54). The authors of this book would not necessarily support Fawcett's (2005) view on this element. With regards to mixing paradigms (or world views), broadly speaking, there are two positions: the purist stance and the a-paradigmatic stance. According to Greene (2007: 68) the purist stance declares,

Paradigms are integrally constituted by sets of interconnected philosophical assumptions (ontological, epistemological and methodological) that must be respected and preserved. The assumptive sets of different paradigms are incommensurable.

and continues,

Paradigmatic assumptions importantly guide and direct practical inquiry decisions. Because the assumptions of different paradigms are incompatible (incommensurable), it is not possible to mix paradigms in the same study.

whereas the a-paradigmatic stance asserts,

Paradigms compose philosophical assumptions and stances regarding reality, knowledge, methodology and values that are logically independent and therefore can be mixed and matched in varied combinations.

So for the authors of this book, the issue is not that the author of a nursing model should uphold the 'purist stance' and have one (and only) underpinning paradigm evident; the issue is more accurately thought of as the need to have a high degree of congruence between any and all paradigms that underpin the model and particular content. Fawcett (1989, 2005: 54) declares that questions to help with determining the models' logical congruence include:

- Does the model reflect more than one world view?
- Does the model reflect characteristics of more than one category of nursing knowledge?
- Do the components of the model reflect logical translation or reformation of diverse perspectives?

By way of an example of a model that perhaps lacks logical coherence, Johnson's (1968) behavioural systems model declares that one of its fundamental values is that society tolerates a wide range of behaviours, yet only the middle section of this continuum of behaviours can be regarded as representative of the so-called cultural norm, and she continues to suggest that the limits of what behaviours are considered acceptable by the healthcare professions, including nurses, will tend to be even narrower than those behaviours considered acceptable by the wider society.

Evidently here Johnson is drawing on key paradigmatic ideas/beliefs about cultural norms and deviance. Yet Johnson (1968) continues to purport that nursing cannot presume to transform the values, beliefs and/or norms of the individuals it serves to those in accordance with the culture of middle-class American society.Thus, nursing and nurses can, according to Johnson (1968), set narrower (and more restrictive) boundaries and limits on what behaviour will be acceptable but at the same time must respect and uphold the individual's inalienable human right to his/her own behavioural norms, values and beliefs.

Generation of theory

Fawcett (1989; 2005) explains how the fourth element is concerned with the extent to which the nursing model leads to the generation of theory; indeed she goes as far as to suggest that at least some theories should be derived from each nursing model. Perhaps this is best expressed (or achieved) by testing some of the propositions pertaining to concepts within the model, and by forming and subsequently testing hypotheses based on these concepts and propositions.

Credibility of the nursing model

Fawcett (1989; 2005) describes how the fifth element is concerned with avoiding uncritical acceptance and therefore focuses on gauging the credibility of the model. Ultimately, Fawcett (2005) argues that evaluating the credibility is necessary to determine which practice settings (and populations) the model would be appropriate for. Once more, the authors note in Fawcett's arguments, evidence of the pivotal relationship between nursing models and their use in clinical practice. Furthermore, a clear implication arising out of Fawcett's (1989, 2005) views is that some models are going to be more relevant (or better suited, some might say) than others; that all conceptual nursing models need not be regarded as equally applicable and/or relevant. Accordingly, if we accept Fawcett's argument, then some nursing models are going to have greater clinical utility than others. However, the authors would argue that the relevance and/or utility of a particular model over another is most likely going to vary according to the specific clinical situations, cultures and scenarios in which they are applied. Thus, limited or low credibility of the model in one nursing scenario need not necessarily indicate the same level of credibility in all other nursing situations. Interestingly, Fawcett (1989, 2005) expands her argument and suggests that the credibility of a nursing model can be gauged by considering the additional criteria of social utility, social congruence and social significance.

Social utility, Fawcett (1989, 2005: 55–56) declares, can be determined by asking the following questions:

- Are education and special skills training required before applying the nursing model in practice? (The need for special skills training and education perhaps indicates a barrier to the model's social utility and thus weakens its credibility.)
- Is it feasible to implement practice protocols derived from the nursing model and related theories? (The feasibility of producing such protocols based on the nursing model is an indicator of increased social utility and thus strengthens its credibility.)
- To what extent is the nursing model actually used to guide nursing research, education, administration and practice? (Extensive and/or increasing evidence of the model's use in these related nursing areas is an indictor of increased social utility and thus strengthens its credibility.)

Social congruence, Fawcett (1989, 2005: 55–56) declares can be determined by asking the following question:

- Does the nursing model lead to nursing activities that meet the expectations of the public and health professionals of various cultures and in diverse geographic regions? (Evidence that the nursing model does not meet this criterion suggests that either the model lacks social congruence and thus credibility, or that the public and other health professionals need to be educated to expect a different kind of nursing.)

Additionally, social congruence, Fawcett (1989, 2005: 55–56) declares can be determined by asking the following question:

- Does application of the nursing model, when linked with relevant theories and appropriate empirical indicators, make important and positive differences in the health conditions of the public?

Once more, where evidence that the nursing model does make important and positive differences to health outcomes in the general public indicates that the model has social significance and thus increased credibility.

Contributions to the discipline of nursing

Fawcett's (1989; 2005) sixth and final element is concerned with the overall contribution of the nursing model; not to be confused with gauging the utility of one model in comparison to another. Not surprisingly, Fawcett (1989, 2005: 57) affirms that this can be determined by asking the following question:

- What is the overall contribution of the nursing model to the discipline of nursing?

Hugh McKenna's (1997) approach to evaluating conceptual nursing models

In his 1997 book *Nursing Theories and Models* McKenna makes the point that many of the approaches for evaluating/critiquing nursing models (and even those designed for evaluating nursing theories) share a great deal of similarity, and that this should not come as a surprise. With apologies to Isaac Newton, each of the designers of these approaches have 'stood on the shoulders' of those theorists who preceded them; their individual approaches to model evaluation are each built upon the seminal contributions of the earlier works of noted epistemologists (e.g. Kuhn, 1962) and therefore, to a greater or lesser extent, all consider the same (or similar) criteria. As a result, McKenna's (1997) approach was an attempt to distil the common elements or criteria that these different approaches have in common, and here we attempt to expand and develop that approach. McKenna's (1997) framework contains five categories, which are listed in *Box 11.2*, and each of these is explored in more detail.

How the model was developed

McKenna (1997) makes very similar remarks to those of Fawcett regarding the consideration or examination of the beliefs and values of the original author of the nursing model. In addition to identifying the philosophical foundations of the model, McKenna argues that there is also value in looking at the geographical origin of the model's author. As we are all, to a greater or lesser extent, a product of our upbringing and background, these formative experiences are likely to influence how we see and make sense of the world (of nursing). A male mental health nurse from the UK whose initial nursing education experiences occurred in the 1980s is very unlikely to have the same world (nursing) view as a female general nurse from the USA whose

---

Box 11.2. Adaptation of McKenna's framework for evaluating nursing theory/models: The five categories to consider

- How the model was developed
- How the model is internally structured
- How the theory might be used
- How the model influences knowledge development
- How the model stands up to testing

---

initial nursing education experiences occurred in the 1950s. Acknowledging and being cognisant of these formative experiences can then help the reader better understand why certain features, philosophical positions and/or clinical emphases are evident in certain models. In addition to the geographical location and clinical background of the model's author, McKenna (1997) makes some enlightening suggestions regarding consideration of the socio-cultural times (and their influence on the author) when the model was created. Indeed, few credible nurse scholars would dispute that one driver for the creation of many early nursing models was the emancipation of nursing as a discrete (and credible) scientific discipline from medicine (Meleis, 1997). (Whether or not nursing has achieved this aim is a highly contested matter of debate, see for example, Cutcliffe and Wieck, 2008.)

How the model is internally structured

According to McKenna (1997) the internal structure of models is a core issue for evaluation and there are (at least) seven criteria within this particular category. These are listed in *Box 11.3*, and then each of these is explored in more detail.

Clarity

Perhaps one of the most important aspects of a theory is its clarity. Clarity may be rated as high or low. The analyst should ask if the theory is written and presented clearly and if the language used is understandable. This refers to or represents semantic clarity. In order to determine or gauge the clarity of the model, you should ask the following questions at a minimum: Are the key terms defined? Are concepts and assumptions implicit? If explicit, are they stated clearly? You should also observe for and note any evidence of tautology (that is any unnecessary repetition and/or excessive 'wordiness'): Is there any evidence of any unnecessary overuse of words? You should also seek to gauge and examine the model's structural clarity. This occurs when

---

Box 11.3. Aspects of the model's internal structure to examine and gauge

- Clarity
- Simplicity or parsimony
- Consistency
- Meta-paradigms
- Adequacy or comprehension
- Soundness or logic of reasoning
- Concepts and propositions

---

the prepositional links between the concepts are clear to the reader and any diagram representing the model can be understood without a great deal of difficulty. If, after trying to understand the model, you still cannot make sense of it, then this suggests it has low clarity.

Simplicity or parsimony

The model should be elegant in its simplicity; that is, the theorist should have decided upon the simplest, most parsimonious format and expression possible, to convey and communicate the model's key theoretical messages. From the outset it should be noted that there are currently no definitive criteria for determining the parsimony of nursing models. Parsimony within the context of the quantitative paradigm on the other hand, has a number of definitions, although it appears to be the case that there is no consensus or agreement about these definitions (Richards, 2002). While some domains of quantitative science appear to have more developed criteria for determining parsimony, see, for example, biogeography, statistics and systematics (Richards, 2002) and even algorithms for calculating parsimony (see Mulaik, 1998), even these domains of science acknowledge the limitations and problems in determining parsimony.

Parsimony refers to a principle, referred to in philosophical literature as Ockham's Razor (Boehner, 1957), wherein the principle is concerned with explaining theory or hypotheses with the fewest number of conceptual elements as possible; of eschewing plurality in favour of simplicity. It is the predilection for the least complex explanation or theory where more than one is available. Indeed, for some the words parsimony and simplicity are synonymous (Hubbard, 2008). Parsimony is also identified as a factor in the field of statistics wherein mathematical models with the lowest number of parameters are preferred to models with higher numbers of parameters. Parsimony also appears in systematics where it is a cladistic optimality criterion (i.e. phylogenetic taxonomy system where organisms are grouped based on their hypothesised phylogeny – or to rephrase, a hypothetical family tree showing ancestral relationships between species) (Poling, 2008). Maximum parsimony in this context then refers to the 'family tree' that requires the fewest number of evolutionary changes to get from species A to species B. So, as with statistics, it is preference for the least complicated 'model' of explanation over a more complicated model (e.g. preference for the model with fewer evolutionary steps). Similarly, in biogeography, parsimony is concerned with the number of migrations and movements of a species. So by examining current geographical distributions of organisms and with reference to the aforementioned phylogenetic tree, the most parsimonious model is one that contains the fewest number of migrations; the lowest amount of total movement.

Hubbard (2008) advances three types of parsimony: epistemological, ontological and linguistic. Epistemological parsimony deals with the *number* of 'things' a theory posits, ontological parsimony deals with the *types* of 'things' a theory posits and linguistic parsimony refers to expressing one's ideas in the shortest sentences possible. Things then, when considering the parsimony of a theory, include concepts, propositions and conceptualisations. Several philosophers have argued that without the presence and influence of this principle, scientific theories and models become needlessly complicated; not least among these philosophers is Popper (1965). Indeed, Popper (1965: 61) declares that, 'it is always advantageous to try the simplest theories first'. Richards (2002) offers similar arguments suggesting that the principle of parsimony requires that the researcher/scholar select the theory/hypothesis that explains the data in the most economical manner.

If nursing wishes its models, practice and research to link appropriately, then models should be easily understood, especially if the model is to gain the attention and 'approval' of hard-pressed, busy clinicians. Clearly, the utility of any model is limited if not thwarted if no-one can understand it; how can a model be used in practice if it cannot be comprehended and understood? This question is equally relevant to the diagrammatic representations that often accompany models. If the diagram is composed of a confusing mixture of geometric lines, different shapes and a variety of arrows, for example, the authors contend that readers will not be impressed. Moreover, busy clinicians are unlikely to have the time to decipher some diagrammatic conundrums. The authors need to add an important caveat here, a realistic conceptualisation of nursing, especially if this is a comprehensive conceptualisation, is likely to be complex, and thus very difficult to express in a simple manner and similarly, very difficult to achieve parsimony. Vaknin (2008) offers similar arguments; he purports that comprehensiveness prevents parsimony.

To obtain a description of the world, which complies with the laws of parsimony, one has to ignore and neglect many elements, facts, and observations. To fully describe the world, however, one would need an infinite amount of assumptions, axioms, theoretical entities, elements, functions and variables. This is anathema to parsimony.

However, the authors would argue that this simplistic Aristotelian view is not completely accurate; the authors assert that the reader is likely to have encountered some models that are clearer, less ambiguous, produce the phenomenological 'Ah ha' or spontaneous validity that Kvale (1996) refers to. Inversely, we suspect that readers may have come across models that are convoluted, unclear, ambiguous, and do not produce the 'Ah ha' or sense of spontaneous validity (just as the authors themselves have). If this is accurate, if some models are more accessible, understandable and applicable than others, then the authors would argue that this might also suggest differences in the degree of parsimony and simplicity of the model.

Consistency

All the elements and components within the model should support one another and be congruent; free from self-contradiction. In other words and for example, a model should not posit one set of actions as being the approach to assessment and then follow this with a different set of assessment-related actions. As with clarity, the reader can then gauge the level of consistency as high or low. Readers should examine the model carefully and note if any inconsistencies are explicit or implicit. Four different types of inconsistency have been identified by Stevens-Barnum (1994) and these are as follows:

- Inconsistency of terms/terminology: definitions of concepts within the model need to be consistent throughout.
- Inconsistency in interpretation: if a model claims to be underpinned by a holistic view of the person, but the model subsequently describes the importance of reducing the person into systems, organs, etc. (i.e. indicative of reductionism and thus the philosophical opposite of holism), then there is significant inconsistency of interpretation evident in the model.
- Inconsistency of principle: again this is concerned with congruence between what the model alleges as important and what using the model actually indicates is important. For example, a model could espouse the importance of self-care and promoting self-care yet if all the nursing actions in the model serve to strip or diminish the individual's personal responsibility, autonomy and/or independence, then there is significant inconsistency of principle evident in the model.
- Inconsistency of method: for example, a theory may have its philosophical origins in phenomenology or existentialism yet the model then includes and advocates for empiricist approaches for its application and testing.

Metaparadigms

Earlier in this book the authors drew attention to the composition of nursing models and made specific reference to Kuhn (1962) and later Fawcett's (1995) key works on metaparadigms (see *Chapter 2*). If one accepts the cogency of Kuhn's and Fawcett's arguments, and clearly the authors of this book do, then the reader should pay particularly close attention to how the metaparadigm components are stated and actualised within the model. The reader should ask: What does the designer of the nursing model say about persons (or people), health, nursing and the environment? Does the designer of the model make these components and the assumptions relating to them explicit, and does the designer of the model emphasise the nature of one paradigm at the expense of the other? Most nursing models tend to include specific and explicit reference to what nursing is (and is not), what health is (and is not), less is included on the nature of persons or people, and most commonly, less still on the nature of the environment. By way of examples, in her original 1859 work, *Notes on Nursing,* Florence Nightingale does make reference to each of the four metaparadigms, although it is accurate to point out that she clearly pays more attention to the nature of people and the environment and the relationship between them; perhaps at the expense of health and nursing. (Interestingly, although Nightingale's (1859) work clearly predates Kuhn's work on metaparadigms, the fact that these metaparadigms are so clearly evident in Nightingale's work perhaps lends further credibility to the legitimacy of Kuhn's ideas.) Similarly, Orem's (1980) model contains a large amount of reference to the nature of nursing as being inextricably linked to self-care, yet by no means the same level of attention or detail is devoted in the model to the nature of the environment – although it is mentioned.

The reader may also find value in examining whether or not the purported relationships between the metaparadigms are stated clearly in the model and if there is a transparent presentation and/or explanation of the beliefs and values and the goals associated with these. At the risk of sounding semantic, the reader may also find value in examining the particular language and expressions used by the designer of the model. For example, if the model refers to 'persons', is this a reference to individual people, patients, potential patients, the person's family, groups of people, communities and/or society at large? When the designer of the model refers to 'nursing', is this a reference to the wider discipline of nursing per se, reference to the so-called art, science or craft of nursing, or is it more specific to the action or particular acts of nursing? When the designer of the model refers to 'environment', is this a reference to the immediate physical environment surrounding the client (and his/her family); is it a reference to the interpersonal atmosphere, relationship and environment constructed between the client and nurse; is it a reference to the meta-physical environment perhaps encapsulated by the term 'milieu' (Bettelheim, 1948/1967; Jones, 1953; Gutheil, 1985); or is it a reference to the wider healthcare setting environment or a more global, wide-scale reference to the wider environment per se? When the designer of the model refers to 'health', is this a reference to the absence of disease or illness, does it refer to a state of well-being, a psycho-social perception; does it refer to or take account of the person's particular stage of development or is it a reference to a state of becoming? What is evident here is that these much used terms have multiple meanings and it is therefore the responsibility of the designer of the model to be clear (and consistent) in the meaning referred to when the terms are used within the model.

Adequacy or comprehension

According to a number of authors (see, for example, Stevens-Barnum, 1994) a model is said to be adequate when it accounts for the subject matter which it purports to deal with. As a result, if a model was designed from experiences in an acute psychiatric ward in the USA, and the designer of the model claimed that its propositions can apply trans-culturally to all nursing situations and scenarios, unless this is an accurate claim, then it indicates an inadequacy; the model may not be trans-culturally transferable and applicable.

By way of examples, the authors here draw on their own, not insignificant, trans-cultural experiences. McKenna, an Irish man by birth, has worked clinically and taught in the UK and has also taught nursing theory at the University of Malawi in southern Arfica. Hyrkas, a Finnish woman by birth, has worked clinically and taught nursing in four different countries including Greece, Canada and the USA. Similarly, Cutcliffe, an English man by birth, has also worked clinically and taught nursing in four different countries including Ireland, Canada and the USA. In each case, the authors have encountered situations where nurses wished to introduce and/or operationalise a particular nursing model, for example Roy or Orem's model in southern Africa (McKenna, 1997) and Barker and Buchanan's tidal (2005) model in Canada. In each case, to a greater or lesser extent and with no disrespect to the authors of those models, the choice of the model was largely driven by the renown and prominence of the author of the model rather than a judicious selection of the model based on its merits and its particular utility within that individual cultural setting. In McKenna's case, the fit between Orem or Roy's model and the cultural nuances of the Malawi nurses was not a strong one; and it would have been better for these nurses to design their own nursing model specific to Malawian nursing. In McKenna's view, this model, with its Malawian-specific concepts, propositions and assumptions, would thus have had the beginnings of adequacy. The same argument, albeit expressed differently, can apply in terms of the particular clinical setting from which the model originated and, the authors would also argue, from which period in time the model was created. Some have argued that Peplau's (1952) model with its origins in American psychiatric nursing may not be particularly adequate for an acute surgical nursing situation, or moreover applicable to a 21st century day surgical unit (given the time frame for establishing and working through the different phases of the relationship). Others have argued that a model such as Peplau's, designed during the 1950s, has limited utility and application to 21st century healthcare settings as a result of sweeping changes in the amount of time nurses spend with clients, the changing nature of the nurses' role, and important changes in healthcare policies. Whereas other authors, such as McNaughton (2005) (and see others in *Chapter 4*) have produced evidence that Peplau's model can be transposed from psychiatry to other clinical settings, albeit with a re-framing of the time periods associated with each phase. Similarly, some have it that while Roy's model (1980, 1996) has particular utility and application to an acute surgical nursing setting, it may not have the same utility or application in a longer-term, care of the adult unit. As a result, it becomes clear that it is important when critiquing and/or evaluating a nursing model to pay attention to its adequacy within the specific cultural, clinical and temporal context in which the model is to be applied.

Soundness or logic of reasoning

A further criterion relating to how the model was formed, McKenna (1997) reminds us, is that of the soundness or logic of reasoning. According to the Wikipedia online encyclopedia (recovered 2009), reasoning is the cognitive process of looking for reasons for beliefs, conclusions, actions or feelings, and logical reasoning can be categorised into three distinguished types: deduction, induction and abduction. Each form of logical reasoning involves a precondition, a conclusion, and a rule that the precondition implies the conclusion. Thus the reader needs to ask of the nursing model: are the internal theoretical conclusions supported by any preceding premises? Here are examples of logical and faulty reasoning:

Logical reasoning example:

- Nursing is an interpersonal process that requires engagement between the nurse and the client (Premise 1).
- People who experience a bereavement sometimes seek to distance themselves from others and sometimes become clients of formal healthcare (Premise 2).
- Nurses need to seek to engage with bereaved clients (Conclusion).

Faulty reasoning

- All clients are actively involved in decision making concerning their care (Premise 1).
- People experiencing some forms of so-called depression can become clients (Premise 2).
- Depressed clients should not be involved in decision making concerning their care (Conclusion).

Concepts and propositions

A well-constructed nursing model should have clearly defined concepts and propositions, particularly as these are the 'theoretical elements or building blocks' upon which the model is built. Further, because propositions refer to the relationships between concepts or, to paraphrase, the way they have been joined together, either poorly defined concepts or weak propositional linkages between the concepts then suggest the model has not been well constructed. Many nursing models will often contain explicit statements as to the nature of the propositions; these in turn can be examined by the reader and subjected to a number of questions such as those put forward by McKenna (1997):

- Do the propositional statements seem valid, logical and relevant to the underlying philosophy of the model?
- Have hypotheses been identified and if so, are they testable, do they have empirical support?
- Have the concepts and propositions been presented in diagrammatic form?

How the model is used

As we have stated previously in this chapter, given that nursing is inescapably a practice-oriented discipline, then nursing models should clearly relate to and be of use in, clinical practice. Notwithstanding the utility that nursing models can and do have as the underpinning to an educational curriculum or research study, the authors of this book concur with Johnson's (1959) pioneering contribution when she considered by what means a model could be analysed. Her comments centred on the model's usefulness for clinical practice and its value to the profession, and that the criteria social utility, social significance and social congruence could be used for this analysis. These criteria find their way into various author's approaches to evaluating nursing models (Fitzpatrick and Whall, 1989; McKenna, 1997; Fawcett, 2005) and we have already covered these in some detail (see above). In addition to Johnson's criteria, McKenna's (1997) approach identifies six other criteria within this particular category. These are listed in *Box 11.4*, and then explored in more detail.

Scope/generality

This criterion relates to how the theory can be applied (to practice/education) and its degree of abstractness. There is perhaps an unstated relationship here, namely, the greater the scope (and generality) of the model, the greater the

---

Box 11.4. Aspects of how the model is used

- Social utility
- Social significance
- Social congruence/acceptance
- Scope/generality
- Guidance for the nursing process
- Accessibility
- Discrimination
- Circle of contagiousness

---

degree of utility (how the model can be used). However, this does not appear to be a direct positive correlation. Grand level nursing models with a higher degree of abstraction are likely to have greater generality since their level of abstraction frees them from restrictions of time, person, culture and space (Glaser, 1998). Nevertheless, because of their grand level and inherent level of abstraction, such models are often difficult to apply and make sense of in practice (or education). Alternatively, a mid-range level nursing model has less abstraction, is less likely to have a broad scope (and generality) yet is much easier to actually apply to practice (or education). Perhaps this is what leads McKenna (1997) to argue that the broader the scope of a model, the greater the possibility that it will be more 'socially congruent'; whereas, the more narrow the scope of the model, the higher its level of 'social utility' will be.

Guidance for the nursing process

Not surprisingly, most nursing models have a very clear connection to the nursing process, or perhaps more accurately to the decision making and problem solving approaches and techniques used in nursing, which are now captured under the term 'nursing process'. McKenna (1997: 233) argues that a nursing model then, 'should bring the nursing process to life'.

If there is merit in this criterion, then the nursing model should speak to each stage or phase of the nursing process: assessment, planning, implementation and evaluation. However, as *Chapters 4–10* indicate, the models we have included in this book are far from being consistent in the attention or focus they each give to all the four phases of the nursing process. Furthermore, some nursing models deliberately eschew some of the terms used in the nursing process and use synonyms and/or paraphrases (see *Chapter 8* on Orem for example). One might expect that more recent models of nursing would perhaps be clearer about their relationship to the nursing process than those earlier models when the nursing process itself was still an emerging idea and not then part of nursing nomenclature.

Accessibility

Clearly, if a nursing model remains inaccessible, then its utility and application to practice (or education) is going to be limited. Very similar to the criteria outlined by Fawcett (1989, 2005), Chinn and Kramer (1995) refer to accessibility as a key criterion in the domain of how the theory is used. They argue that a model needs empirical indicators that reflect its concepts in order for it to be tested (in the 'real world'). While the authors of this book concur that a model that has been subjected to some testing in the real world can be more accessible (assuming the tests indicate that the model does work), we would not necessarily agree that a model that has not been subject to testing has no utility. Throughout history the scientific academe has produced many models which, at the time, there was a lack of sophisticated instrumentation and/or 'methodological know how' to test them. However, as such advances occurred, some models were subsequently subjected to testing and were shown to be accurate (see, for example, Parker's, 1959, discovery of the 'solar wind').

Discrimination

Nursing is a discrete discipline whose view of phenomena may differ in perspective compared to that of other disciplines. You should seek to find out if the theory has the capacity to differentiate between those who provide nursing from other health professionals and from informal family care givers. This is an essential quality in any applied discipline that borrows many of its scientific ideas from other disciplines. If a nursing model does not show how nursing is unique compared to other disciplines, then one might wonder if it is a nursing model at all.

Circle of contagiousness

In the UK we have imported several American nursing models and Meleis (1997) would refer to this geographical spread of a model, not directly influenced by its author, as the 'widening circle of contagiousness'. In your evaluation you may wish to note whether the model has been altered in its trans-cultural, cross-frontier journey and who was directly responsible for its introduction into your country. Within which specialty areas is it being used? How is it being used?

How the model influences knowledge development

According to McKenna (1997), nursing models can be evaluated in terms of how they influence knowledge development, in terms of theory generation and importance (*Box 11.5*).

Theory generation

Nursing models should be examined to gauge whether or not the theory has the potential to stimulate the generation of other nursing theory. For example, the discerning reader will be able to detect the influence of earlier written models in models written latterly (see for example, the influence of Rogers', 1980, in Fitzpatrick and Whall's, 1982, theory.) And such model-to-model influence is entirely in keeping with cumulative models of knowledge generation and/or what has been termed the 'incremental change of routine science' (see Gamota, 2006). Alternatively, grand level models can (should) lead to the development of mid-range and practice theories.

Importance

Chinn and Kramer (1995) argue that whether or not a model influences knowledge development can be considered by gauging if the model is forward looking; does it speak to the advancing of nursing practice, does the model serve as the underpinning theoretical framework for nursing research studies, or does it serve as the framework for nursing curricula? The essence of this area for consideration is whether or not (in the view of the reader/reviewer) the model will help or hinder the development of nursing knowledge.

How the model stands up to testing

There has been a great deal written about the necessity of testing or evaluating models in order to provide evidence of the utility and accuracy (or validity) of their concepts and assumptions (see for example, Fawcett, 2005). Even the most ardent supporter of nursing academia and products of nursing science would have to admit that few (if any) nursing models have been subjected to such evaluation, although there is some such evidence in existence.

One of the most important contributions in this area is Silva's (1986) work on examining the amount and type of work to test the assumptions and propositions within the model. Silva (1986) found that these types of study were rare. Drawing together 62 model testing studies published in the

---

Box 11.5. How the model influences knowledge development

- Theory generation
- Importance

American nursing literature between 1952 and 1985, and applying a rigid set of seven criteria, Silva (1986) reported three categories of studies that focus on testing nursing models (see *Box 11.6*).

Similarly, in an attempt to determine how many purported nursing research studies actually tested nursing theory, Moody et al (1988) undertook a more comprehensive study and examined 720 studies of nursing practice research. (Although it is important to point out here that nursing research should not always be concerned with theory testing; that theory-inducing studies are just as valuable, the pre-occupation with quantitative, positivist, i.e. theory testing, research notwithstanding.) Moody et al (1988) report finding that less than 5% of the studies examined actually tested concepts, hypotheses or propositions from the nursing models. Also in the 1980s, Cheryl Beck (1985) found that few nursing research studies actually tested any nursing models, findings once more supported by Allen and Hayes' (1989) review.

Having identified two approaches to evaluating nursing models, both of which highlight how problematic such endeavours are, it is necessary to situate current attempts within the contemporary epistemological climate; one that is perhaps best captured by the phrase 'evidence-based' or 'evidence-informed' practice.

Conceptual nursing models and the movement towards evidence-based or evidence-informed practice

It would be remiss of the authors of this book to include a chapter on evaluating and critiquing nursing models without paying any attention to the particular epistemological climate in which much (if not all) of contemporary health care is currently operating: that of the so-called evidence-based (or more accurately evidence-informed) practice movement. In order to understand

---

Box 11.6. Silva's categories of research studies that focus on testing nursing models

- Category One: Minimal use. Accounting for roughly one third of all such studies, these papers use the nursing model as the underlying theoretical framework but do not test, explicitly, any part of the model
- Category Two: Insufficient use. Accounting for almost half (and thus the majority) of all such studies, these papers contain elements of the nursing model, and are used to inform and organise the research instruments
- Category Three: Adequate use. Accounting for the minority of all such studies, these papers contain a comprehensive test of the model, meeting all of Silva's (1986) seven criteria

the processes and practices of evaluating and critiquing nursing models in this era of 'evidence-based or evidence-informed' practice it is necessary to examine the key components of evidence-based practice, namely, research; evidence and critiquing/critical reading of the literature.

What is research?

The often quoted definition of research provided by the UK Department of Health (1994: 37) asserts that research is:

Rigorous and systematic enquiry conducted on a scale and using methods commensurate with the issue to be investigated, and designed to lead to more generalised contributions to knowledge.

Research then involves a systematic search for knowledge, and healthcare research is thus concerned with uncovering knowledge that is important (and useful) for health practitioners. As intimated in the Department of Health's definition, there exists a wide range of research methods and methodologies, which are broadly grouped together under two paradigms: the quantitative and the qualitative. Each paradigm is concerned with the uncovering of new knowledge, however, the type of knowledge produced and the way the researchers go about uncovering this knowledge is different within each paradigm. Kerlinger (1986), one of many advocates of the quantitative approach to research, asserts that the way to truth is through rigorous research, involving the identification of variables within hypotheses and subjecting them to experimental manipulation. Here 'hard evidence' is required in order to be certain that something is or is not true. To Kerlinger, this approach is at the peak of a hierarchy of how to know; further down were less respectable ways of knowing, including 'tenacity', 'authority' and 'a priori'. The end result of each of these ways of knowing is knowledge; what differs is how the knowledge is acquired. Kerlinger has great respect for knowledge gained through the scientific quantitative method and less for knowledge gained through what he perceives as more subjective approaches. However, the importance of qualitative research, what Kerlinger would describe as 'subjective', and the different forms of evidence will be explored in more detail below.

The historical dominance of quantitative research within healthcare

Examination of the research undertaken within medicine and healthcare indicates a clear historical emphasis on quantitative studies. Significantly, at first, medicine was only interested in quantitative studies and in particular, randomised controlled trials (RCTs) and RCTs were regarded in the UK as the 'gold standard' of robust clinical enquiry. However, since the early 1990s some of those working within medicine and healthcare have recognised the need to use the large amount of other forms of research and evidence at its disposal to inform its work. Nevertheless, reviews of RCTs became essential during this time (Haynes et al, 1996; Roth and Fonagy, 1996) because it was impractical for practitioners to read everything that has been published for themselves. Not only that, but also not all the RCTs report the same results (Chalmers and Altman, 1995). Hence, you may have a situation where half of a group of research projects indicate that treatment X is the best, while the other half suggest that treatment Y is of better value. If the practitioner only reads the first group of projects he or she would be inclined to use treatment X, and likewise for those only reading papers which recommended treatment Y. Four things, therefore, occurred during the 1990s to deal with the massive increase in available research material.

- The development of models to enable individuals critically to appraise or review single and groups of literature papers (Greenhalgh, 1997b; NHSE, 1999).
- The development of models to undertake systematic reviews of large amounts of literature (Cullum, 1994; NHS Centre for Reviews and Dissemination, 1996; Hek et al, 2000).
- The development of databases and review libraries that would make available completed reviews carried out by panels of clinical and research experts in the field (Lefebvre, 1994; Brazier and Begley, 1996).
- The development for researchers of guidelines that would inform the design and management of robust clinical trials (Medical Research Council, 2000).

In theory, these four activities should provide a framework to ensure that practitioners know how to review literature and how to access reviews of large amounts of literature. Researchers should have a better understanding of how to carry out and report on their work. The problem with this is that it assumes that all staff are able to access these skills, or acquire them while they are undertaking their professional training and education, which patently is not the case. Furthermore, up until the 1990s, it was also (wrongly) assumed that the only critically sound research was that carried out using quantitative methods of enquiry for both medicine and nursing, yet this was patently not the case (Sackett et al, 1997; Ward et al, 1999). As authors have pointed out, much within (nursing and) other healthcare is not susceptible to quantitative research methods (see Smith, 1998).

The movement towards a more pluralistic approach

As a result, pressure for the inclusion of qualitative research studies and other forms of evidence to be included within the scope of evidence-based practice came from several sources including professional academia, the social sciences, clinical psychology, nursing, and medicine, particularly psychiatry. Their reasoning was obvious and contained two main arguments. The first was that quantitative research examines known phenomena, e.g. one therapy against another, one or both of which have already been in use and are being compared to establish effectiveness against each other, or the statistical outcome value of a drug used to reduce symptoms for a recognised diagnostic entity such as one of the forms of schizophrenia. However, qualitative researchers suggest that for this research to take place, the entity itself has to be placed in context otherwise it is unclear just what the drug or therapy is acting upon. Thus, as Dodd (2001) argues, indicating the need for preliminary exploratory, descriptive, contextual, phenomenological and anthropological studies, i.e. those which describe entities, are the domain of qualitative research.

The second, and perhaps more important, argument was that qualitative research is not simply used to describe contexts for entities. There are known phenomena that in themselves are not susceptible to quantitative processes, e.g. belief structures, feelings, interactions, etc. (and an argument has been suggested which purports that much of nursing may be invisible or immeasurable and thus, not accessible using quantitative methods). Thus qualitative methods are required in order to understand the nature and complexity of these phenomena. Healthcare is inescapably concerned with human interactions and the ability of patients (people) to develop personal strategies for living. True, for some there is a major role for surgery, medication and other forms of physical therapy in this work, but essentially it is people-intensive and deals with emotions, thoughts and adaptability. Similarly, as we have already described, such care is being delivered in ever changing environments and, increasingly, community settings, very often those of the patient's own home. For research to make sense of these entities and for that research to be of value to practitioners wanting to implement it into their own work it has to be environment- and people-focused. Qualitative researchers argue that these types of services, and the personal work that they undertake, are the domains of their methods.

Further evidence of embracing methodological pluralism

Even the most cursory examination of the extant methodological literature, and perhaps more significantly, the systematic review literature, will show that methodological pluralism is becoming the latest orthodoxy. Inextricably linked to this development is the growing recognition and valuing of findings from qualitative studies. Moreover, the criticisms that qualitative studies can sometimes be 'isolated' and parochial in nature is being addressed by means of a number of processes, not least the development of methods for systematic review of qualitative studies and the increasing attention given to qualitative meta-synthesis (see, for example, the work emerging from the various international Cochrane Centres, such as Popay et al, 2008; Pluye et al, 2008; Florence et al, 2008). At the present moment, it would be epistemologically premature to assert that developments in qualitative meta-synthesis are robust and without methodological controversy. Nevertheless, such intellectual tussles are not only useful, they are necessary. The emerging findings from these endeavours are, however, compelling and worthy of examination. Before so doing, it is necessary to remind ourselves of the nature of the generalisable findings that qualitative studies aspire to.

Qualitative researchers do not seek to generalise their findings in the same way that a quantitative researcher might. That is, they do not seek nomothetic generalisations relating to universal laws and absolute 'truths'. They do seek, however, to produce idiographic or naturalistic generalisations. That is, generalisations about and drawn from cases (Sandelowski, 1997). Generalisations that are drawn from purposeful samples that have experience of the 'case' are thus applicable to similar 'cases', questions, and problems, irrespective of the similarity between the demographic group. In psychiatric/mental health nursing studies, for example, each 'case' of nursing will bear a clear resemblance to psychiatric/ mental health nursing as a 'whole' and any related, similar 'cases'. Thus, a process that is identified in one setting, group or population (i.e. one case), can be similarly experienced by another related setting, group or population. For example, a Grounded Theory concerned with inspiring hope induced from a sample of nurses is likely to be generalisable to, and bear similarity to, any population that shares the process of hope inspiration.

Work on the systematic review of qualitative studies using the Joanna Briggs Institute Qualitative Assessment and Review instrument (Florence et al, 2008) perhaps illustrates the nature of idiographic generalisable findings. Individual researchers from the UK, Spain, USA, Canada, Thailand, Hong Kong, China and Australia independently produced a meta-synthesis of qualitative studies, with 18 pairs of reviewers from diverse cultures and contexts. The results of the meta-synthesis exercise were analysed to identify the degree to which inter-reviewer agreement/consensus was achieved between these 18 pairs. In spite of the differences in background, the similarity in meaning of the synthesised findings across the participant pairs was striking. There was remarkable consistency within and between groups. Other methodological work is occurring which attempts to combine and synthesise quantitative meta-analyses and qualitative meta-syntheses (see, for example, Popay et al, 2008; Pluye et al, 2008). Accordingly, while it remains the case that quantitative methods still hold the dominant position within nursing research (especially if one adopts an international perspective and examines the funding/publication patterns in different countries), there are very clear signs that there is movement within the academic community towards methodological pluralism; and a parallel recognition that the nursing and healthcare research academe needs both paradigms in order to achieve the most complete understanding possible.

What is evidence? The different forms of evidence

As indicated in the previous section, some authors regard the findings or results produced from a quantitative research study to be 'hard evidence'. Appleby et al (1995), for example, intimate that evidence is reliant on the existence of (quantitative) research findings. However, as we similarly indicated in the previous section, it is important to acknowledge that a more pluralistic perspective exists. In their often quoted work, Sackett et al (1996) provide a definition of evidence-based practice that does not specifically mention quantitative research. They see it as 'the conscientious, explicit and judicious use of current best evidence in making decisions about the care of individual patients'. Similarly, McKibbon and Walker (1994) offer an even less rigid definition of evidence-based practice, representing it as 'an approach to healthcare that promotes the collection, interpretation and integration of valid, important and applicable patient-reported, clinician-observed, and research-derived evidence'.

As a consequence of accepting more pluralistic views of the nature of evidence, and perhaps as a way to explain the apparent contradictions in definitions of evidence-based practice (McKenna et al, 2000), hierarchies of evidence have been suggested, such as the hierarchy described in *Box 11.7*.

It needs to be acknowledged that such hierarchies of evidence are by no means universally accepted. An alternative, and well-accepted, view posits that research methods within quantitative and qualitative paradigms can be regarded as a 'tool kit'; a collection of methods that are purposefully designed to answer specific questions and discover particular types of knowledge. To attempt to place these designs (and the evidence they produce) into some artificial and linear hierarchy only serves to confuse and obfuscate. If what is needed to answer a particular problem (e.g. the comparison of the therapeutic effects of two drugs) is a meta-analysis of the current studies in one particular area, then for that particular problem, that is clearly the best form of evidence. Concomitantly, if what is required to answer a particular problem (e.g. what is the lived experience of suffering violent incidents) is

---

Box 11.7: Hierarchy of evidence

- Level 1: meta-analysis of a series of randomised controlled trials
- Level 2: at least one well-designed randomised control trial
- Level 3: at least one controlled study without randomisation
- Level 4: non-experimental descriptive studies
- Level 5: reports or opinions from respected authorities

Based on Muir-Gray (1997)

---

deep, thorough, sophisticated understanding, then for that particular problem, that is clearly the best form of evidence.

Certainly there has been a gradual acceptance among the scientific community within healthcare that there is a definite role for both methodological forms (Mueser et al, 1998; Fenton, 2000; Popay et al, 2008; Pluye et al, 2008; Florence et al, 2008). Additionally, it is also recognised that it is necessary to undertake research that uses both quantitative as well as qualitative research and there is a growing trend for such approaches within healthcare (Gournay et al, 2001; Lester, 2002; Goldney, 2002; Cutcliffe, 2005). Greenhalgh (1999) described this as the dissonance between the 'science' of objective measurement and the 'art' of clinical proficiency and judgement. She attempted to integrate these different perspectives into clinical methods, albeit for psychiatry although the approach was certainly consistent with nursing.

In addition to the evidence produced by qualitative research studies, the definitions of Sackett et al (1996, 1997) and McKibbon and Walker (1994), and Muir Gray's (1997) hierarchy, each allude to additional forms of evidence, namely, reports (grey literature), opinions from experts/respected authorities, conference presentations, results from audits, continuous quality improvement initiatives and, importantly, patient reported information. What such an extensive list clearly indicates is that the absence of formal research findings (from quantitative or qualitative studies) does not mitigate against evidence-based decisions. As McKenna et al (2000: 40) state:

What is required is the best evidence available – not the best evidence possible.

Mixed method and qualitative evaluation of nursing models: A possible approach

Greene's excellent 1997 book *Mixed Methods in Social Inquiry* reminds us that the later half of the 20th century saw a growing discontent with the prevailing orthodoxy within social science; an increasing recognition that confining social science to observable, measurable phenomena constrained and weakened such research. As a result, the last 30 years have seen more and more mixed methods designs in social science evaluation studies (Greene, 2007). Interestingly, even though there is little or no disagreement that nursing falls squarely under the banner of 'social science' and, with that, nursing models (and the science of nursing models) are *ipso facto* matters of social science, very little mixed methods research has been undertaken to evaluate models. At the risk of getting drawn into tired methodological debates, what is noticeably absent are qualitative studies and qualitative components within mixed method designs. This is particularly puzzling to the authors given that, as we have previously stated, there are well-documented problems in positivistic, empirical evaluation of nursing models, particularly given the abstract and general nature of the propositions in conceptual (nursing) models makes them not amenable to direct observation or empirical testing. Therefore, the next section of this chapter offers some preliminary remarks concerning how qualitative evaluation of nursing models might occur.

Phenomenological approaches to evaluating nursing models

Phenomenological approaches are concerned with describing and understanding particular phenomena as lived experience. They involve the rigorous, critical and systematic study of 'essences', the purpose of which is to explicate the structure or essence of the lived experience of a phenomenon in the search for the 'unity meaning', which is the identification of the essence of the phenomenon, and its accurate description through everyday lived experience. Accordingly, nursing models might, at least in part, be evaluated by means of accessing, describing and understanding the lived experiences of practitioners (and educators) who use a nursing model.

While a range of methods exist under the broad banner of phenomenology (see Colaizzi, 1976; Gadamer, 1976; Van Manen, 1997; Giorgi, 1985), and these methods draw upon a range of phenomenological philosophy (e.g. Sartre, 1943; Heidegger, 1962; Merleau Ponty, 1962; Husserl, 1964) each asserts that phenomenology is inductive. There is utility in understanding nursing behaviours as a result of the nurse's life, his or her experiences and the situated contextual meaning that the person attributes to these experiences (Heideggar, 1962). According to Morse and Field (1995), phenomenological researchers ask questions of participants in order to answer the question: 'What is it like to have a certain experience?' So with respect to nursing model evaluation, researchers might ask questions such as, 'What is it like to have your particular experience of using or attempting to use the nursing model?' Examples of such questions are included in *Box*

11.8. Phenomenologists draw upon the 'life world' of the participants as the primary source of data, however, this can be supplemented by literature, poetry, art or artefacts (Sandelowski, 1994). Further, these participants are drawn upon 'purposefully' as they can speak to the lived experience in the greatest depth, and accordingly, phenomenological researchers use 'purposeful' rather than random sampling selection. Thus for a phenomenological evaluation of the nursing model, the researcher would have to purposefully sample practitioners who have had specific experience of using and/or implementing the nursing model in question. The product of a phenomenological evaluation of a nursing model study should be a text, and an accurate description (and in some cases interpretation) of the experiences of using the model.

Ethnographic approaches to evaluating nursing models

Ethnographic research in healthcare-related matters, including the evaluation of nursing models, has its roots in cultural anthropology (Morse and Field, 1995). Ethnographic studies of nursing models then need to be informed by the concept of culture (Boyle, 1994). Further, while acknowledging the variations within the different types of ethnography, typically all ethnographies attempt to be holistic, reflexive and contextual (Boyle, 1994). Ethnographies attempt to account for human behaviours from the 'emic' perspective; from the perspective of those who are on the inside, those who participate in the behaviour. Ethnographers attempt to elucidate the particular beliefs, nuances, idiosyncrasies and practices that exist within certain cultures, yet these understandings have to be obtained by the researcher observing and perhaps participating in the context (and culture) in which they occur. Accordingly, the ethnographer will use a variety of data collection methods. Most often some form of observation (participatory or otherwise) and field note taking will occur, and this can and is augmented by additional methods.

Ethnographic evaluations of nursing models then would need to ask questions such as, 'This community of nurses has introduced nursing model X into their clinical area, how has the introduction of the model altered and/or affected how members of this community and culture activity construct their 'new cultural world'? What is it like for nurses working in this new nursing model-influenced community? What beliefs, nuances, idiosyncrasies, and behaviours exist within this community and culture that may influence the acceptance/rejection, utility/failure of this newly introduced nursing model? How are the beliefs, behaviours and practices affected by the introduction of nursing model X?' Thus, ethnographers wish to determine if and how practitioners can actively

---

Box 11.8: Examples of questions used in a phenomenological study of the lived experiences of suicidal Alberta males

- Can you describe your experience of attempting to use nursing model 'X' as you live(d) with it?
- Can you try and describe the experience from the inside as it were, almost like a state of mind: your feelings, your mood, your emotions, your thoughts?
- Can you focus on a particular example or incident of using the nursing model; can you describe specific events, particular happenings?
- Could you focus on an example of the experience of using the nursing model that stands out for its vividness?
- Could you describe how your body felt at that time you were using the nursing model, how things smelled, how they sounded?

(adapted from Van Manen, 1997)

---

shape their lives within these cultures, such as a culture that includes a newly introduced nursing model. Importantly, in place of studying people, ethnographers learn from people and this allows for the 'emic' perspective; the 'insiders' view' to emerge (Boyle, 1994). The product of an ethnography will involve description, but Morse and Field (1995) argue it should move beyond description. The ethnographer needs to identify and explicate social patterns and observed conduct. According to Geertz (1973), the product of an ethnographic study is typically, thick description, the search for shared meaning within the cultural norms, the patterned behaviour that is indicative of the culture, and the cultural context. Accordingly, ethnographic evaluations of nursing models ought to produce thick descriptions of the culture, the patterned behaviour following the introduction of the nursing model.

Grounded Theory approaches to evaluating nursing models

Glaser and Strauss (1967) first developed the method(ology) of Grounded Theory and published this in their now seminal text, *The Discovery of Grounded Theory: Strategies for Qualitative Research*. Its basic and central theme is generating theory from data that is systematically obtained from social research. Consequently, Grounded Theory is an inductive process. It is a method(ology) for developing or inducing a theory that should provide clear enough categories and hypotheses that explain and aid understanding of the basic (psycho)social process being studied. As a result, a Grounded Theory evaluation of a nursing model should provide an explanatory theory of how the nursing model enhances nurses' care; how the nursing model affects, influences and drives the very processes of nursing as it is carried out in the care setting(s).

In Grounded Theory, as data are collected, the process of constant comparative analysis occurs whereby each item or label of data is compared with every other item or label. Thus, data collection, sampling and data analysis each occur simultaneously. Further, the methodological choices of where to go for the next data and what questions to ask are driven by the emerging theory not by an a priori research design decision; such a process is called 'theoretical sampling' (Glaser, 1978). This process of theoretical sampling means that participants need to be selected according to their knowledge and experience of the (psycho)social process under study. Thus, in evaluating nursing models, a Grounded Theory study would need to sample nurses who were actively involved in introducing the model or have worked on the care unit after the introduction of the model.

The theory of how the nursing model affects and influences care would then be seen to originate from the 'ground level', from the social world from where the data originate. As Stern (1994) suggests, Grounded Theory scientists construct theory from the data rather than applying a theory constructed by someone else from another data source. Thus the theory remains connected to, or grounded in the data, and in that way grounded in reality; the specific reality of where the data originated from; in the case of nursing model evaluation, the specific reality of the nursing model as it is used in real practice.

Concluding remarks

In the 'era of evidence' the *carte blanche* adoption or introduction of any nursing model into clinical practice seems ill advised at best and inappropriate at worst. The authors would argue that in the epoch of 'evidence-informed practice', the adoption or introduction of a nursing model for one's clinical area ought to be accompanied by some form of evaluation. Interestingly, there appears to be little or no disagreement in the extant literature on this matter; even though measuring the effectiveness of nursing models is no simple task. This may particularly be the case if researchers restrict themselves to using only quantitative designs. Encouragingly though, for each of the nursing models featured in this book, the authors located some evaluation evidence; although, as pointed out previously, these evaluations either used the model only as the theoretical underpinning to a study, or as a theoretical guide to certain practice development initiatives, or measured one/some proposition or concept contained with a model. What the authors found to be noticeably absent from this evaluation literature was mixed methods design evaluations and/or evaluations that utilised a variety of qualitative methods (the preponderance of case studies notwithstanding). While such approaches to evaluation of nursing models appear to be atypical at the moment, it is important to note that mixed method evaluation of other complex social phenomena has occurred and is well documented (see Greene, 2007).

For readers then who concern themselves with evaluating nursing models in the contemporary epistemological climate of evidence-based (or evidence-informed) practice, a key issue becomes: What constitutes evidence in our evaluation of the nursing model? Do we limit our evidence to positivistic numerical data obtained from deductive, quantitative studies? Do we limit ourselves to narrative data obtained from inductive, case study-based qualitative evaluations? Or do we seek to obtain and consider multiple different types of evidence?

In the view of the authors of this book, an evaluation of a nursing model in these contemporary times clearly needs to draw on various forms of evidence; it needs to acknowledge the credibility, utility and 'validity' of multiple forms of evidence and use this evidence in a meaningful way. While no doubt beset with methodological problems and epistemological positions to reconcile, the problem of evaluating a nursing model is not insurmountable. Nurses who wish to undertake such evaluations might find specific value in mining the extant literature that focuses on evaluating complex (and sometimes abstract) social phenomena such as the programme evaluation literature in social sciences (see Greene, 2007). It seems so obvious as perhaps to be tautological of the authors but we would argue that any introduction of a nursing model to practice ought to be followed by a multi-method evaluation; thereby confirming (or refuting) the utility of the model for that specific area of practice. Furthermore, if the results are published and placed in the public domain, they add to the body of evidence that other practitioners might access when they are considering the evidence base of any given model. Lastly, and by no means least, any evaluation of a nursing model would be incomplete and severely lacking in meaning, in the view of the authors, if it does not include a significant component that focuses on whether and how the model influences clinical practice.

References

Allen MN, Hayes P (1989) Models of nursing: Implications for research in nursing. In Akinsanya J (Ed) *Recent Advances in Nursing*. Churchill Livingstone, Edinburgh

Appleby J et al (1995) *Acting on the Evidence*. Research paper. National Association for Health Authorities and Trusts London

Barker P, Buchanan P (2005) *The Tidal Model. A Guide for Mental Health Professionals*. Brunner-Routledge, London and New York

Beck CT (1985) Theoretical Frameworks. Cited in Nursing Research from January 1974 to June 1985 *Nurse Educator* **10**(6): 36–8

Bettelheim B (1948/1967) *The Empty Fortress*. Free Press, New York

Boehner P (1957) (trans) *Ockham: Philosophical Writings*. Thomas Nelson and Sons, London

Boyle J (1994) Style of ethnography. In Morse JM (Ed) *Critical Issues in Qualitative Research Methods* (pp 159–85). Sage, Thousand Oaks

Brazier H, Begley CM (1996) Selecting a database for literature searches in nursing: MEDLINE or CINAHL? *Journal of Advanced Nursing* **24**(4): 868–75

Chalmers I, Altman DG (Eds) (1995) *Systematic Reviews*. BMJ Publishing Group, London

Chinn P, Kramer MK (1995) *Theory and Nursing: A Systematic Approach*. CV Mosby, St Louis

Cody WK (1999) Middle-range theories: Do they foster the development of nursing science? *Nursing Science Quarterly* **12**: 9–14

Colaizzi PF (1975) Psychological research as the phenomenologist views it. In Valle R, King M (Eds) *Existential Phenomenological Alternatives for Psychology* (pp 48–71). Oxford University Press, Oxford

Cullum N (1994) Critical reviews of the literature. In Hardey M, Mulhall A (Eds) *Nursing Research. Theory and Practice*. Chapman and Hall, London

Cutcliffe JR (2005) Towards an understanding of suicide in First Nation Canadians Crisis: *Journal of Crisis Intervention and Suicide Prevention* **26**(3): 141–5

Cutcliffe J, Wieck L (2008) Salvation or damnation: Deconstructing nursing's aspirations to professional status. *Journal of Nursing Management* **16**: 499–507

Department of Health (1994) *Working in Partnership: The Report from the Mental Health Review Team*. HMSO, London

Dickoff J, James P (1968) A Theory of theories: A position paper. *Nursing Research*   **17**(3): 197–203

Dickoff J, James P, Wiedenbach E (1968) Theory in a practice discipline: 1 Practice oriented discipline. *Nursing Research* **17**(5): 415–35

Dictionary.com (2009) *Definition of critique*. Available from: http://dictionary. reference.com/browse/critique

Dodd T (2001) Clues about evidence for mental health care in community settings – assertive outreach. *Mental Health Practice* **4**: 10–14

Fawcett J (1989) *Analysis and Evaluation of Conceptual Models of Nursing* (3rd Edn). FA Davis, Philadelphia

Fawcett J (1993) *Analysis and Evaluation of Nursing Theories*. FA Davis, Philadelphia

Fawcett J (2005) *Contemporary Nursing Knowledge: Analysis and Evaluation of Nursing Models and Theories* (2nd Edn). FA Davis, Philadelphia

Fenton WS (2000) Evolving perspectives on individual psychotherapy for schizophrenia *Schizophrenia Bulletin* **26**: 47–72

Fitzpatrick JJ, Whall AL (1982) *Conceptual Models of Nursing: Analysis and Application*. 1st Edn, Appleton & Lange, Norwalk

Fitzpatrick JJ, Whall AL (1989) *Conceptual Models of Nursing: Analysis and Application*. 2nd Edn, Appleton & Lange, Norwalk

Florence Z, Schulz T, Pearson A (recovered 2008) Inter-reviewer agreement: An analysis of the degree to which agreement occurs when using tools for the appraisal, extraction and meta-synthesis of qualitative research findings *Cochrane Collaboration* From: http://www.cochrane.org/colloquia/abstracts/melbourne/O-69.htm

Freud SJ (1915–17) *Introductory Lectures on Psychoanalysis*. Penguin, Harmondsworth (Reprinted 1979)

Gadamer HG (1976) *Philosophical Hermeneutics* (Linge DE trans and Ed) University of California Press, Los Angeles

Gamota G (2006) *Towards a science-based framework for developing science metrics*. Available from: http://www.wren.network.net/events/2003

Geertz C (1973) *The Interpretation of Cultures*. Basic Books, New York

Glaser BG, Strauss AL (1967) *The Discovery of Grounded Theory: Strategies for Qualitative Research*. Aldine, Chicago

Glaser BG (1978) *Theoretical Sensitivity: Advances in the Methodology of Grounded Theory*. Sociology Press, Mill Valley, California

Glaser BG (1992) *Basics of Grounded Theory Analysis: Emerging Versus Forcing*. Sociology Press, Mill Valley, California

Glaser BG (1998) *Doing Grounded Theory: Issues and Discussions*. Sociology Press, Mill Valley California

Giorgi A (1985) Sketch of a psychological phenomenological method. In: Giorgi A (Ed) *Phenomenology and Psychological Research* (pp 8–22). Duquesne University Press, Pittsburgh

Goldney RD (2002) Qualitative and quantitative approaches in Suicidology: Commentary. *Archives of Suicide Research* **6**(1): 69–73

Gournay K, Plummer S, Gray R (2001) The dream team at the institute. *Mental Health Practice* **4**: 15–17

Greene JG (2007) *Mixed Methods in Social Inquiry*. Wiley, San Francisco

Greenhalgh T (1997a) How to read a paper: Papers that report drug trials. *British Medical Journal* **315**: 480–3

Greenhalgh T (1997b) *How to Read a Paper*. BMJ Publishing Group, London

Greenhalgh T (1999) Narrative-based medicine in an evidenced-based world. *British Medical Journal* **318**: 323–5

Gutheil T (1985) The therapeutic milieu: Changing themes and theories. *Hospital and Community Psychiatry* **36**: 1279–85

Haynes R, McKibben K, Kanani R (1996) *Systematic Reviews of RCTs of the Effects of Patient Adherence and Outcomes of Interventions to Assist Patients to Follow Prescriptions for Medications Cochrane Library* (Updated 30 August 1996) BMJ Publications, London

Hek G, Langton H, Blunden G (2000) Systematically searching and reviewing literature. *Nurse Researcher* **7**(3): 40–57

Henderson V (1966) *The Nature of Nursing: A Definition and Its Implications for Practice, Education, and Research*. Macmillan, London

Heidegger M (1962) *Being and Time*. Harper Row, New York

Hubbard J (1995) *Parsimony and the mind*. Available from:http://www.tk421.net/essays/simple.html. [Last accessed April 2008]

Husserl E (1964) *The Idea of Phenomenology*. Alston W Nakhikan G (trans) Nijhoff, The Hague

Jarrrett J (1988) *ŒNietzsches Zarathrustra: Notes of the seminar given in 1934–39 by CG Jung*. Bolinger Series Princeton University Press, New Jersey

Johnson D (1959) The nature of a science of nursing. *Nursing Outlook* 7: 291–4

Johnson DE (1968) Theory in nursing: Borrowed and unique. *Nursing Research* 17(3): 206–9

Johnson DE (1987) Evaluating conceptual models for use in critical care nursing practice. *Dimensions of Critical Care Nursing* 6: 195–7

Jones M (1953) *The Therapeutic Community*. Basic Books, New York

Kerlinger FNB (1986) *Foundations of Behavioural Research* (3rd Edn) Holt, Rinehart and Winston, New York

Kuhn T (1962) *The Structure of Scientific Revolutions* (1st Edn) University of Chicago Press, Chicago

Kvale S (1996) *Interviews: An Introduction to Qualitative Research Interviewing*. Sage, Thousand Oaks

Lefebvre C (1994) The Cochrane Collaboration: The role of the UK Cochrane Collaboration in identifying evidence. *Health Libraries Review* 11

Lester D (2002) Qualitative versus quantitative studies in psychiatry: Two examples of cooperation from suicidology. *Archives of Suicide Research* 6(1): 15–18

McKenna HP (1997) *Nursing Theories and Models*. Routledge, London

McKenna HP, Cutcliffe JR, McKenna P (2000) Evidence-based practice: Demolishing some myths. *Nursing Standard* 14(16): 39–42

McKibbon KA, Walker CJ (1994) Beyond ACP Journal Club: How to harness Medline for therapy problems. *Annals of Internal Medicine* 121(1): 125–7

McNaughton DB (2005) A Naturalistic test of Peplau's Theory in home visiting. *Public Health Nursing* 22(5): 429–38

McWilliam CL, Godfrey B, Stewart M, Sangster J, Mitchell J, Cohen, I (2003) Evolving the delivery of acute services in the home. *Home Health Care Services Quarterly* 22(1): 55–74

Marris J, Lowry LW (2006) Nursing theory and practice: Connecting the dots. *Nursing Science Quarterly* 19(1): 44–50

Medical Research Council (2000) *A Framework for Clinical Trials of Complex Health Interventions*. Medical Research Council, London

Meleis AI (1997) *Theoretical Nursing: Development and Progress* (3nd Edn). Lippincott, Philadelphia

Merleau-Ponty M (1962) *Phenomenology of Perception* (Smith C trans) Humanities Press, New York

Moody LE, Wilson M, Smyth K, Schwartz R, Tittle M, VanCott M (1988) Analysis of a decade of nursing practice research. *Nursing Research* 37: 374–9

Morse JM, Field PA (1995) *Qualitative Research Methods for Health Professionals* (2nd Edn) Thousand Oaks, London

Mueser K, Bond G, Drake R et al (1998) Models of community care for severe mental illness: A review of research on case management. *Schizophrenia Bulletin* **24**: 37–74

Muir Gray JA (1997) Evidence Based Health Care. Churchill Livingstone, Edinburgh

Mulaik SA (1998) Parsimony and Model Evaluation. *Journal of Experimental Education* **66**: 266–72

National Health Service: Centre for Reviews and Dissemination (1996) *Undertaking Systematic Reviews of Research on Effectiveness. CRD Report No 4.* Centre for Reviews and Research on Effectiveness, York

National Health Service Executive (1999) *Critical Appraisal Skills Programme.* NHSE Anglia and Oxford

Nightengale F (1859) *Notes on nursing: What it is and what it is not* (reprinted 1980) Churchill Livingstone, Edinburgh

Orem DE (1980) *Nursing: Concepts and Practice* (3rd Edn), McGraw Hill, New York

Parker EN (1959) Dynamics of the interplanetary gas and magnetic fields. *Journal of Astrophysics* **128**: 664

Pearson A (1992) Knowing nursing: Emerging paradigms in nursing. In Robinson K, Vaughan B (Eds) *Knowledge for Nursing Practice*. Butterworth Heinemann, Oxford

Peplau HE (1952) *Interpersonal Relations in Nursing*. GP Putnam & Sons, New York

Pluye P, Grad R, Levine A, Nicolau B (2008) Understanding divergence of quantitative and qualitative data (or results) in mixed methods studies. *International Journal of Multiple Research Approaches* **3**(1): 58–72

Poling J (1997) *What is parsimony, anyway?* From:http://www.dinosauria.com/jdp/misc/parsimony.htm [Last accessed April 2008]

Popay J, Roberts H, Sowden A, Petticrew M, Britten N, Arai L, Roen K, Rodgers M (recovered 2008) *Developing methods for the narrative synthesis of qualitative and quantitative data in systematic reviews of effects*. From: http://www.york.ac.uk/inst/crd/projects/narrative-synthesis.htm [last accessed 10 August 2009]

Popper K (1965) *Conjectures and Refutations: The Growth of Scientific Knowledge*. Harper & Row, New York

Richards R (2002) Kuhnian values and cladistic parsimony. *Perspectives on Science* **10**(1): 1–27

Rodgers BL (2005) *Developing Nursing Knowlwedge: Philosophical Traditions and Influences*. Lippincott Williams & Wilkins, Philadelphia

Rogers ME (1980) *An Introduction to a Theoretical Basis of Nursing* (2nd Edn). FA Davis & Co, Philadelphia

Roth A, Fonagy P (1996) *What Works for Whom? A Critical Review of Psychotherapy Research*. Guilford Press, New York

Roy C (1980) The Roy Adaptation Model. In Riehl JP, Roy C (Eds) *Conceptual Models for Nursing Practice*. Appleton-Century-Crofts, New York

Roy C (1996) The Roy Adaptation Model. In Riehl JP, Roy C (Eds) *Conceptual Models for Nursing Practice*. Appleton-Century-Crofts, New York

Sackett DL, Rosenberg W, Muir-Gray J et al (1996) Evidence-based medicine: What it is and what it isn't. *British Medical Journal* **312**: 71–2

Sackett DL et al (1997) *Evidenced-based medicine: How to Practice and Teach EBM*. London, Churchill Livingstone

Sandelowski M (1994) Towards a poetic for qualitative inquiry. In Morse JM (Ed) *Critical Issues in Qualitative Health Research* (pp 46–63). Sage, Thousand Oaks, London

Sandelowski M (1997) 'To be of use': Enhancing the utility of qualitative research. *Nursing Outlook* **45**(3): 125–32

Sartre JP (1943) In Blackham HJ (1986) *Six Existentialist Thinkers* (pp 58–79). Routledge London

Silva MC (1986) Research testing nursing theory: The state of the art. *Advances in Nursing Science* **9**(1): 1–11

Smith P (1998) *Nursing Research: Setting New Agendas*. London, Arnold

Stern PN (1994) Eroding grounded theory. In Morse JM (ed) *Critical Issues in Qualitative Research Methods* (pp 210–23). Sage, London

Stevens-Barnum BJ (1994) *Nursing Theory: Analysis, Application and Evaluation* (4th Edn). Lippincott, Philadelphia

Vaknin S (2008) *Parsimony: The fourth substance*. From: http://samvak.tripod. com/parsimony.html [Last accessed April, 2008]

Van Manen M (1997) *Researching Lived Experience: Human Science for Action Sensitive Pedagogy*. State University of New York Press, New York

Ward MF, Cutcliffe J, Gournay K (1999) *A Review of Research and Practice Development Undertaken by Nurses, Midwives and Health Visitors to Support People with Mental Health Problems*. United Kingdom Central Council for Nurses, Midwives and Health Visitors, London

Wikipedia Online Encyclopedia (2009) *Logical Reasoning*. From: http:// en.wikipedia.org/wiki/Logical_reasoning [Last accessed January 2009]

Index